CONTENTS

4

INTRODUCTION

What is the Hamilton Beach Breakfast Sandwich Maker?

Let's be perfectly clear: The Hamilton Beach Breakfast Sandwich Maker is not a gourmet, high-tech, fancy cooking tool for super-serious cooks. Not at all. What it is, though, is fun. And it's well-built and sturdy, considering what it's designed to do. And it works just like it's supposed to. The whole idea is to make a breakfast sandwich like the ones from fast-food restaurants. You could certainly do that with normal cooking equipment—a toaster, frying pans, egg rings—but that's really not the point. This gadget makes the process a little more user-friendly. Or cooking-challenged friendly. Because this isn't really like cooking. It's a simple assembly process that just about anyone could manage. The idea is that you start with the bottom of a muffin, add meat, cheese, or vegetables on top, close that section and put an egg on the next layer, and put the top piece of bread on top of the egg. Close it up, and in about five minutes, the egg is cooked, the bread is toasted, and everything is very hot. Slide the bottom out from under the egg, and there's a complete sandwich

Why Do You Need It?

There is a lot to love about this breakfast sandwich maker, but the things that most users find to be the most beneficial are:

Breakfast in Under 5 Minutes... Without Actually Making It

No more rushing the most important meal of the day, no more gobbling down unhealthy pre-made and packaged choices. With this amazing appliance, you can enjoy your breakfast in under 5 minutes, without having to stir, sauté, or flip in front of the stove. While the Hamilton Beach Breakfast Sandwich Maker does its job, you get to prepare your coffee, fix your hair, get dressed or do whatever it is your doing on a hectic morning. All you need to do is simply assemble the ingredients, set the timer, and that's it!

One-Dish Meal

Okay, let's say you want to enjoy a breakfast sandwich, but do not own the Hamilton Beach Breakfast Sandwich Maker. You will need to toast the buns/bread, fry the egg separately, maybe even warm your pre-cooked meat, and then assemble the ingredients. That will require that you use a toaster or a roasting pan, another pan for the fried egg, a spatula, etc. Which leaves you with a bunch of dishes for washing. Who has time for that in the morning? This appliance will both toast your eggs, warm the ingredients, and fry the eggs at the same time. And you will only have one dish for washing.

Evenly Cooked

When preparing breakfast sandwiches the traditional way, it is pretty hard to achieve a consistent crispiness and even temperature. Why? Because you don't do it all at once. You will need to separately fry your eggs, toast your breads, melt your cheeses, etc. Some will be cooked more than the others, the bread may go cold while you whip up your eggs, etc. This appliance though, does it all at ones.

Your job is only to assemble the ingredients and it will cook the egg perfectly, toast the bread to ideal crispiness, melt the cheese, and leave you with a center that is delectably warm. You cannot achieve this evenness another way. And you get it all in under 5 minutes which is why it is said that the Hamilton Beach Breakfast Sandwich Maker makes one high-class breakfast.

Affordable
Unlike other fancy cooking appliances that costs hundreds of dollars, the Hamilton Beach Breakfast Sandwich Maker will not break your bank. In fact, you can get it in just $24.99. And the best part? You don't have to buy two appliances so that you and your loved one can enjoy warm breakfast together. Hamilton Beach offers a Dual Breakfast Sandwich Maker that allows you to cook two separate sandwiches at the same time. And the price? Just $39.99.

You Can Make Omelets
But, besides for being great for making sandwiches, the Hamilton Beach Breakfast Sandwich Maker is also a unit that will help you perfectly fry eggs and cook omelets as well. Just add the eggs without any bread or other additions, and you will have a first-class omelet in just 3-4 minutes.

How Does It Work?

If you've been wondering whether the appliance works as smoothly as in the commercial – yes, you can be sure it does. The process couldn't be more straightforward – you just pile up your ingredients and that's it:
1.Arrange half bun at the bottom.
2.Add a slice of cheese and/or some meat that is pre-cooked (ham, bacon, sausage, etc.)
3.Crack an egg into the barrier.
4.Top with the other half of bun.
5.Close and cook for 4-5 minutes.

Additional Tips for Best Results

Here are some additional tips that will up your cooking with the Hamilton Beach Breakfast Sandwich Maker:
● Use round breads, buns, and bagels for best results. You can trim the edges of a normal loaf bread to fit perfectly, but that is not a requirement. You can also just place the bread as it is and smash a bit to fit. It might get darker around the edges, but it will still be perfectly toasted.
● Do not smoosh. Place the lid gently and do not press on it; it is not a panini maker. Pressure is not required for ideal cooking here.
● It is all in the timing. For perfectly cooked breakfast, find the perfect cooking time. Set a kitchen timer or do it on the phone, but make sure to cook for the ideal time.
● Taking a peek is allowed. If you are not sure whether your sandwich is ready or not, simply open the lid and take a peek, just like you'd do with your oven.
● Always use mittens when opening the cover of the unit. The surface is hot and there can be steam escaping so getting burn is a possibility you need to be aware of.

CLASSIC BREAKFAST SANDWICH RECIPES

1.   Mediterranean Sandwich

Servings: 4
Cooking Time: 20minutes
Ingredients:
- 4 rolls, ciabatta, split
- 4 oz. Feta cheese, crumbled
- 24 oz. spaghetti or marinara sauce, divided
- 7 ½ oz. artichoke hearts, marinated, quartered and then chopped
- 2 Tomatoes, sliced
- 1 lb. Deli Turkey sliced thinly

Directions:
1. Spread 2 tbsp. marinara sauce on 4 roll halves.
2. Top the halves with cheese, turkey, tomato artichokes and again cheese. Spread 2 tbsp. Sauce and place the turkey. Top with the second roll hales.
3. Cook on the sandwich maker for 5 minutes.
4. Serve and enjoy!

2.   Tomato Basil Flatbread

Servings: 1
Cooking Time: 5 Minutes
Ingredients:
- 1 small round flatbread
- 1 tsp. olive oil
- Salt and pepper to taste
- 1 thick slice ripe tomato
- 4 fresh basil leaves
- 1 slice fresh mozzarella cheese
- 1 large egg

Directions:
1. Preheat the breakfast sandwich maker.
2. Place the round flatbread inside the bottom tray of the sandwich maker.
3. Brush the flatbread with the olive oil and sprinkle with salt and pepper.
4. Top the flatbread with the slice of tomato, basil leaves and mozzarella cheese.
5. Slide the egg tray into place and crack the egg into it. Use a fork to stir the egg, just breaking the yolk. Close the sandwich maker and cook for 4 to 5 minutes until the egg is cooked through
6. Carefully rotate the egg tray out of the sandwich maker then open the sandwich maker to enjoy your sandwich.

3.   Portabella And Spinach Croissant

Servings: 1
Cooking Time: 5 Minutes
Ingredients:
- 1 croissant, sliced
- 1 tsp. olive oil
- 1 cup baby spinach
- 1 tbsp. grated parmesan cheese
- 1 clove garlic, minced
- 1 portabella mushroom cap
- Salt and pepper to taste
- 1 large egg

Directions:
1.   Heat the olive oil in a small skillet over medium heat. Stir in the garlic and cook for 1 minute.
2.   Add the spinach and cook for 2 minutes, stirring, until just wilted. Remove from heat and stir in the parmesan cheese.
3.   Preheat the breakfast sandwich maker.
4.   Place half of the croissant, cut-side up, inside the bottom tray of the sandwich maker.
5.   Top the croissant with the spinach mixture and the portabella mushroom cap. Sprinkle the mushroom with salt and pepper to taste.
6.   Slide the egg tray into place and crack the egg into it. Use a fork to stir the egg, just breaking the yolk.
7.   Place the second half of the croissant on top of the egg.
8.   Close the sandwich maker and cook for 4 to 5 minutes until the egg is cooked through.
9.   Carefully rotate the egg tray out of the sandwich maker then open the sandwich maker to enjoy your sandwich.

4.   Egg White Sandwich With Spinach And Goat's

Servings: 1
Cooking Time: 5 Minutes
Ingredients:
- 1 Whole Wheat English Muffin
- 2 Egg Whites
- 1 ounce Goat's Cheese
- 1 tbsp chopped Spinach
- 1 tbsp chopped Pepper
- Salt and Pepper, to taste

Directions:
1.   Preheat and grease the sandwich maker.
2.   Whisk the egg whites and season with some salt and pepper.
3.   Cut the muffin in half.
4.   Place one half in the bottom of the unit, with the cut-side up.
5.   Top with the cheese, spinach, and pepper.
6.   Lower the cooking plate and ring and pour the egg whites inside.
7.   Top with the second half of the muffin, this time with the cut-side down.
8.   Close the unit and cook for 5 minutes.
9.   Rotate clockwise to open and transfer to a plate with a plastic or wooden spatula.
10. Serve and enjoy!
Nutrition Info: Calories 255 Total Fats 7.7g Carbs 29.5g Protein 19.5g Fiber 5.5g

5.   Corned Beef And Cabbage Panini

Servings: 2
Cooking Time: 8 Minutes
Ingredients:
- 1 cup thinly sliced green cabbage
- 1 Tablespoons. olive oil
- ¼ teaspoon. table salt
- Freshly ground black pepper
- 1 teaspoon. yellow mustard seeds
- 2 Tablespoons. unsalted butter, softened
- 4 1/2-inch-thick slices rye bread with caraway seeds
- 1 Tablespoons. grainy mustard, more to taste
- 12 thin slices (6 oz.) corned beef
- 6 thin slices (3 oz.) Muenster cheese
- ¼ cup water

Directions:
1.   Mix the water, cabbage, olive oil, mustard seeds, salt, and pepper in a saucepan, heat on medium-high heat until water boils. Once boiling lower heat to medium-low heat, cover, allow the mixture to cook for 10 to 15 minutes, stirring every once in a while. Remove the cabbage from the saucepan, and set aside any remaining water in the pan.
2.   Butter one side of each piece of bread and place mustard on the other side. Top two pieces of bread, mustard side up with corned beef, then cabbage, and finally cheese. Top with the remaining pieces of bread, butter side up.
3.   Cook the sandwiches for 6 to 8 minutes on medium heat, and make sure to flip halfway through. The bread should be brown, and the cheese should be melted.

6.   Provolone Baby Mushroom And Caramelized Onion Panini

Servings: 5
Cooking Time: 4 Minutes

Ingredients:

- 2 tablespoons unsalted butter
- 2 tablespoons olive oil
- 1 and 1/2 large onions (or 2 medium) sliced into 1/4 inch thick slices
- 1 tablespoon sugar
- 1/4 teaspoon thyme
- 2 tablespoons minced garlic (I used 1 and 1/2)
- 1 teaspoon Worcestershire sauce
- 8 oz. fresh baby Bella mushrooms, sliced into 1/4 inch thick slices
- 1/2 teaspoon black pepper
- salt to taste
- 1/4 - 1/2 teaspoon red pepper flakes (or more to taste)
- 1 teaspoon flour
- 1/4 cup mushroom broth (or beef broth)
- 2 tablespoons minced parsley
- 5 - 1 oz. slices provolone cheese, cut in half
- 10 slices of fresh French bread
- Olive oil

Directions:

1.   Heat a big skillet on medium heat, making sure it's hot before adding any ingredients. Put in the olive oil and butter, and allow the butter to melt. Then put in the onions and allow them to cook for 5 minutes. Mix in the sugar and cook for an additional 15 minutes. Mix in the Worchester sauce, garlic, and thyme, and allow the mixture to cook for 2 more minutes before mixing in the mushrooms. Cook for 10 minutes before mixing in the red and black pepper along with the flour. Slowly mix in the broth 1 tablespoon at a time, waiting until it's been absorbed before adding another. After you've added all of the broth and it's been absorbed, remove it from the heat and mix in the parsley.

2.   Place a layer of cheese on 5 pieces of bread, then the vegetable mixture, and then another layer of cheese. Top with the remaining slices of bread. Brush the olive oil on both the top and bottom of the sandwiches.

3.   Cook the Panini on medium high heat for 3 to 4 minutes, flipping halfway through. The bread should be toasted, and the cheese should be melted.

7.   Classic Italian Cold Cut Panini

Servings: 2
Cooking Time: 6 Minutes
Ingredients:
- 1 12 inch hoagie rolls or the bread of your choice
- 1 tablespoon olive oil
- 2 ounces Italian dressing
- 4 slices provolone cheese
- 4 slices mortadella
- 8 slices genoa salami
- 8 slices deli pepperoni
- 4 slices tomatoes
- 2 pepperoncini peppers, chopped

Directions:
1. Slice the rolls in half and then cut it open.
2. Lightly coat the outside of the roll with olive oil using a brush.
3. Brush the inside each piece of bread with the dressing. Then top the bottom pieces of bread with cheese. Add the mortadella, salami, tomatoes and pepperoncini's
4. Cook the Panini on medium heat for 6 minutes, flipping halfway through. The bread should be brown, and the cheese should be melted.

8.   Peach Basil Croissant

Servings: 1
Cooking Time: 4 Minutes
Ingredients:
- 1 small croissant, sliced in half
- 1 – 2 Tbsp. cottage cheese
- 2 tsp. peach jam
- Fresh sliced peaches
- Basil leaves
- Dash of cinnamon

Directions:
1. Spread cottage cheese and peach jam on both croissant halves. Place one half into the bottom ring of breakfast sandwich maker, jam side up. Place peach slices and basil leaves on top. Sprinkle with cinnamon.
2. Lower the cooking plate and top ring; top with other croissant half. Close the cover and cook for 3 to 4 minutes or until sandwich is warmed through. Remove from sandwich maker and enjoy!

9.   Lamb Panini With Mint And Chili Chutney

Servings: 4
Cooking Time: 55 Minutes
Ingredients:
- ¾ cup Chili Chutney
- 2 teaspoon fresh mint, finely chopped
- 1 teaspoon wholegrain mustard
- 2 tablespoons sour cream or cream cheese
- Salt and freshly ground black pepper
- 4 Panini rolls or olive Ciabatta rolls, cut in half
- 4-8 slices roast lamb
- ½ cup caramelized red onion
- ½ cup feta cheese, crumbled
- 1½ cup arugula

Directions:
1.   Combine the chutney, mint, mustard, sour cream, and pepper. Allow it to rest for 15 minutes
2.   Spread the chutney mixture on the inside part of both halves of the rolls. Brush the other side of the bread with olive oil. Put a layer of onions on the bottom half of the roll, then lamb, arugula, and then feta, and top with the other half of the roll.
3.   Cook the sandwiches for 6 minutes on medium heat, and make sure to flip halfway through. The bread should be nicely toasted and the cheese should be melted.

10.   Eggs Florentine Biscuit

Servings: 1
Cooking Time: 5 Minutes
Ingredients:
- 1 slice multigrain bread
- 1 large egg
- 2 tbsp. plain nonfat yogurt
- ¼ tsp. Dijon mustard
- ½ cup baby spinach
- 1 tbsp. minced yellow onion
- 1 tsp. olive oil

Directions:
1.   Heat the oil in a small skillet over medium heat. Add the onion and spinach and stir well.
2.   Cook for 2 minutes, stirring, until the spinach is just wilted. Set aside.
3.   Preheat the breakfast sandwich maker.
4.   Place the piece of bread inside the bottom tray of the sandwich maker.
5.   Whisk together the yogurt and mustard in a small bowl then brush over the piece of bread.
6.   Top the bread with the cooked spinach and onion mixture.
7.   Slide the egg tray into place and crack the egg into it. Use a fork to stir the egg, just breaking the yolk.
8.   Close the sandwich maker and cook for 4 to 5 minutes until the egg is cooked through.
9.   Carefully rotate the egg tray out of the sandwich maker then open the sandwich maker and enjoy your sandwich.

11.   Turkey Salsa Melt

Servings: 1
Cooking Time: 4 Minutes
Ingredients:
- 2 ounces leftover Turkey, chopped up nicely
- 1 English Muffin
- 1 tbsp Salsa
- 1 ounce shredded Cheese by choice
- 1 tsp chopped Celery

Directions:
1. Preheat and grease the sandwich maker.
2. Cut the muffin in half and place one half on top of the bottom ring, with the cut-size up.
3. Combine the turkey and salsa and place on top of the muffin.
4. Add the celery on top and sprinkle the cheese over.
5. Lower the top ring and add the second half with he cut-size down.
6. Close and cook for 4 minutes.
7. Carefully open the lid and transfer to a plate.
8. Serve and enjoy!

Nutrition Info: Calories 410 Total Fats 22g Carbs 21g Protein 20g Fiber 0.9g

12.   Chocolate Croissant

Servings: 1
Cooking Time: 3 Minutes
Ingredients:
- 2 ounces Chocolate, chopped
- 1 Croissant
- 1 tsp Heavy Cream

Directions:
1. Preheat the sandwich maker and grease it with some cooking spray.
2. Cut the croissant in half and place one half on top of the bottom ring, with the cut-side up.
3. Arrange the chocolate pieces on top and sprinkle with the heavy cream.
4. Lower the top ring and add the second croissant part, with the cut-side down.
5. Cook for 3 minutes.
6. Open carefully and transfer to a plate.
7. Serve and enjoy!

Nutrition Info: Calories 283 Total Fats 14g Carbs 32g Protein 6g Fiber 1.8g

13.   Ham And Relish Melt

Servings: 1
Cooking Time: 5 Minutes
Ingredients:
- 2 slices white or multigrain bread
- Butter
- 1 Tbsp. sweet pickle relish
- 1 slice ham
- 1 slice cheddar cheese
- 1 egg
- Sea salt and pepper

Directions:
1.   Butter the outside of each slice of bread. Spread relish on the inside of each slice. Place one slice into the bottom ring of breakfast sandwich maker, relish side up. Place ham and cheddar cheese on top.
2.   Lower the cooking plate and top ring; crack an egg into the egg plate and pierce to break the yolk. Season with sea salt and pepper. Top with other slice of bread.
3.   Close the cover and cook for 4 to 5 minutes or until egg is cooked and cheese is melted. Carefully remove sandwich with a rubber spatula.

14.   Tomato And Pepper Omelet With Mozzarella

Servings: 1
Cooking Time: 4-5 Minutes
Ingredients:
- 2 Eggs
- 1 ounce shredded Mozzarella Cheese
- 2 Tomato Slices, chopped
- 1 ½ tbsp chopped Red Pepper
- 1 tsp chopped Parsley
- ¼ tsp Onion Powder
- ¼ tsp Garlic Powder
- Salt and Pepper, to taste

Directions:
1.   Preheat and grease the sandwich maker.
2.   Beat the eggs and season with onion powder, garlic powder, and salt and pepper.
3.   Stir in the parsley.
4.   Pour half of the eggs inside the bottom ring.
5.   Top with the mozzarella, chopped pepper and tomatoes.
6.   Lower the top ring and cooking plate and pour the rest of the eggs into the plate.
7.   Close and cook for about 4 to 5 minutes.
8.   Rotate the handle clockwise, lift to open, and transfer the omelet to a plate.
9.   Serve and enjoy!
Nutrition Info: Calories 240 Total Fats 26g Carbs 4.2g Protein 19.3g Fiber 0.7g

15.   Orange Dream Donut

Servings: 1
Cooking Time: 5 Minutes
Ingredients:
- 1 medium glazed donut, sliced in half lengthwise
- Cream cheese
- Orange marmalade
- 1 tsp. orange zest
- 1 egg
- Sea salt and pepper

Directions:
1.   Spread cream cheese and orange marmalade on both donut halves. Place one half into the bottom ring of breakfast sandwich maker, jam side up. Sprinkle with orange zest.
2.   Lower the cooking plate and top ring; crack an egg into the egg plate and pierce to break the yolk; sprinkle with sea salt and pepper. Top with other donut half.
3.   Close the cover and cook for 4 to 5 minutes or until egg is cooked through. Gently slide the egg plate out and remove donut with a rubber spatula.

16.   Ham And Cheese Egg Biscuit Sandwich

Servings: 1
Cooking Time: 5 Minutes
Ingredients:
- 1 Biscuit, halved
- 2 Red Pepper Rings
- 1 Egg
- 1 Ham Slice
- 1 slice American Cheese
- Salt and Pepper, to taste

Directions:
1.   Preheat the sandwich maker and grease with some cooking spray.
2.   When the green light appears, place the bottom half of the biscuit in the bottom ring.
3.   Top with the cheese, ham, and pepper rings.
4.   Lower the cooking plate and crack the egg into it. Season with some salt and pepper.
5.   Add the top biscuit half on top and close the appliance.
6.   Cook for 5 minutes.
7.   Open carefully by sliding clockwise and transfer with plastic spatula to a plate.
8.   Serve and enjoy!

Nutrition Info: Calories 270 Total Fats 15.5g Carbs 14g Protein 17.7g Fiber 0.5g

17.   Peach Caprese Panini

Servings: 1
Cooking Time: 4 Minutes
Ingredients:
- 1 French deli roll, split
- 1 ½ teaspoon balsamic vinegar
- 2 slices mozzarella cheese
- 1 small heirloom tomato, sliced
- 4 fresh basil leaves
- olive oil
- 1 small peach, sliced

Directions:
1.   Sprinkle the balsamic vinegar on the inside of both pieces of bread. Brush the outside of both pieces of bread with olive oil
2.   Place one of the mozzarella slices on the bottom piece of bread, then the peaches, then the tomatoes, and top with the other piece of cheese. Place the other piece of bread on top of the cheese.
3.   Cook the Panini on medium heat for 3 to 4 minutes, flipping halfway through. The bread should be toasted, and the cheese should be melted.

18.   Chicken Pesto Sandwich

Servings: 2
Cooking Time: 30minutes
Ingredients:
- 4 tbsp. Olive oil
- 2 chicken breasts, skinless and boneless
- 1 tsp. Oregano, dried
- ¼ tsp. Pepper fakes
- Black pepper and salt to taste
- 2 rolls, ciabatta
- ¼ cup of Pesto
- 1 sliced Tomato
- 4 oz. Mozzarella, fresh, sliced

Directions:
1.   Turn on medium heat and place a skillet. Add 2 tbsp. olive oil. While the oil heats season with chicken with black pepper, salt, pepper flakes, and oregano. Cook the chicken 7 minutes on each side. Set aside.
2.   Now slice the rolls and spread pesto. Top with mozzarella, chicken, and tomato. Spread pesto again. Top with the other half of the roll.
3.   Heat the sandwich press and coat with 2 tbsp. oil. Add one sandwich and press. Cook 5 minutes. Repeat with the second roll.
4.   Serve and enjoy!

19.   Creamy Brie Pancake Sandwich

Servings: 1
Cooking Time: 5 Minutes
Ingredients:
- 2 frozen pancakes
- 1 tablespoon raspberry jam
- 1 ounce Brie, chopped
- 1 large egg

Directions:
1.   Preheat the breakfast sandwich maker.
2.   Place one of the pancakes inside the bottom tray of the sandwich maker and spread the raspberry jam on top.
3.   Sprinkle the chopped brie on top of the pancake.
4.   Slide the egg tray into place and crack the egg into it.
5.   Top the egg with the other pancake.
6.   Close the sandwich maker and cook for 4 to 5 minutes until the egg is cooked through.
7.   Carefully rotate the egg tray out of the sandwich maker then open the sandwich maker and enjoy your sandwich.

20.   Sauerkraut Sandwich

Servings: 1
Cooking Time: 5minutes
Ingredients:
- 1 Hard roll, cut in half
- ½ cup Sauerkraut
- Sliced Bratwurst, cooked
- 2 oz. Swiss Cheese, shredded

Directions:
1.   Cut the hard roll in half.
2.   On one-half place the sauerkraut, bratwurst, and cheese. Place the second half of the roll.
3.   Place on the sandwich maker and press for 5 minutes.
4.   Serve and enjoy!

21. Tomato, Egg And Avocado

Servings: 1
Cooking Time: 5 Minutes
Ingredients:
- 1 croissant, sliced
- 2 slices ripe tomato
- ¼ ripe avocado, pitted and sliced
- 1 slice Swiss cheese
- 1 large egg
- 1 tablespoon sliced green onion
- 2 teaspoons half-n-half

Directions:
1. Preheat the breakfast sandwich maker.
2. Place half of the croissant, cut-side up, inside the bottom tray of the sandwich maker.
3. Top the croissant with the tomato and avocado, then top with the slice of Swiss cheese.
4. Whisk together the egg, green onion and half-n-half in a small bowl.
5. Slide the egg tray into place and pour the egg mixture into it.
6. Top the egg with the other half of the croissant.
7. Close the sandwich maker and cook for 4 to 5 minutes until the egg is cooked through.
8. Carefully rotate the egg tray out of the sandwich maker then open the sandwich maker and enjoy your sandwich.

22. Meat Lover's Biscuit

Servings: 1
Cooking Time: 5 Minutes
Ingredients:
- 1 buttermilk biscuit, sliced
- 2 slices Canadian bacon
- 1 pork sausage patty, cooked
- 1 slice deli ham
- 1 large egg

Directions:
1. Preheat the breakfast sandwich maker.
2. Place half of the biscuit, cut-side up, inside the bottom tray of the sandwich maker.
3. Arrange the slices of Canadian bacon, sausage and ham on top of the biscuit half.
4. Slide the egg tray into place and crack the egg into it.
5. Top the egg with the other half of the biscuit.
6. Close the sandwich maker and cook for 4 to 5 minutes until the egg is cooked through.
7. Carefully rotate the egg tray out of the sandwich maker then open the sandwich maker and enjoy your sandwich.

23.   Chicken And Bacon Paprika Sandwich

Servings: 1
Cooking Time: 4 Minutes
Ingredients:
- 1 ounce ground Chicken
- 1 ounce cooked and crumbled Bacon
- ¼ tsp smoked Paprika
- 2 Red Pepper Rings
- 1 slice of Cheese
- 1 tsp chopped Onion
- 2 tsp Dijon Mustard
- 1 small Hamburger Bun

Directions:
1. Preheat the sandwich maker until the green light appears and grease it with some cooking spray.
2. Cut the hamburger bun in half and brush the insides with the mustard.
3. Place one half with the mustard-side up, on top of the bottom ring.
4. Add the chicken and bacon and sprinkle the paprika over.
5. Top with the pepper, onion, and add the cheese on top.
6. Lower the top ring and finish it off by adding the second bun, placed with the mustard-side down.
7. Close the lid and cook for 4 minutes.
8. Open the lid with mittens, and carefully transfer to a plate.
9. Serve and enjoy!

Nutrition Info: Calories 298 Total Fats 13g Carbs 21g Protein 23.5g Fiber 5.5g

24.   Huevos Rancheros On Tortilla

Servings: 1
Cooking Time: 4 Minutes
Ingredients:
- 1 Mini Wheat Tortilla
- 1 tsp chopped Red Pepper
- 1 Egg
- 2 tsp chopped Onion
- 1 tbsp Beans
- 2 tsp Salsa
- ¼ cup shredded Cheddar Cheese
- Salt and Pepper, to taste

Directions:
1. Preheat and grease the sandwich maker.
2. With a cookie cutter, cut out the tortilla if needed so it can fit inside the sandwich maker.
3. Whisk the egg in a bowl or directly in the cooking plate, and season with salt and pepper.
4. Stir in the onion and red pepper.
5. Place the tortilla into the bottom ring.
6. Place the beans and cheese on top.
7. Lower the cooking plate and pour the egg inside.
8. Close the unit and cook for 4 minutes.
9. Rotate clockwise to open and transfer to a plate, carefully, with a plastic spatula.
10. Top with the salsa.
11. Serve and enjoy!

Nutrition Info: Calories 360 Total Fats 21g Carbs 16g Protein 18g Fiber 2.5g

25. Cheddar Sandwich With Prosciutto

Servings: 1
Cooking Time: 3 ½ Minutes
Ingredients:
- 2 slices White Bread
- 2 slices Cheddar Cheese
- 1 Prosciutto Slice
- 1 tbsp Butter

Directions:
1. Preheat the sandwich maker and grease it with some cooking spray.
2. Trim the bread slices or cut in a circle with a cookie cutter, to make sure they fit inside.
3. Spread the butter onto the slices.
4. When preheated, place one bread circle in the bottom ring with the butter-side up.
5. Top with the prosciutto and cheese.
6. Add the second bread slice with the butter side down.
7. Close and let the sandwich cook for about 3 ½ minutes.
8. Open by sliding out the cooking plate clockwise.
9. Transfer to a plate and enjoy!

Nutrition Info: Calories 495 Total Fats 27g Carbs 39.7g Protein 27.5g Fiber 6g

26. Mortadella Ricotta Sandwich

Servings: 1
Cooking Time: 5minutes
Ingredients:
- 2 tbsp. Ricotta
- A dash of salt
- Black pepper to taste
- ½ tsp. Thyme, chopped
- ½ tsp. Parsley, chopped
- 2 bread slices (Italian crusty bread)
- 4 Slices of Mortadella

Directions:
1. Combine the ricotta, salt, black pepper, parsley, and thyme. Mix well and spread on the two pieces of bread.
2. On one of the slices layer the mortadella slices and place the second slice on top.
3. Grill on the sandwich maker for 5 minutes and serve.

27. Thai Peanut Peach Panini With Basil

Servings: 1
Cooking Time: 8 Minutes
Ingredients:
- 2 tbsp. creamy natural peanut butter
- 1 tbsp. agave or maple syrup
- 1/2 tbsp. soy sauce or tamari
- 1/2 tbsp. lime juice
- 2 slices good sandwich bread
- 1 small or 1/2 large peach sliced thin
- 2 tbsp. fresh basil leaves
- 1-2 tsp. olive oil
- Butter, softened

Directions:
1. Mix together the first 4Ingredients:using a whisk. If the sauce is too thick you can thin it out with a small amount of water. The sauce will natural thin when it's grilled.
2. Spread a large amount of the peanut sauce on what's going to be the inside pieces of bread. Layer the peaches and basil on the peanut sauce side of one of the pieces of bread, and then top with the other. Spread the butter on the top and bottom of the sandwich
3. Cook the Panini on medium heat for 6 to 8 minutes, flipping halfway through. The bread should be brown, and the cheese should be melted.

28.   Avocado And Mixed Vegetable Panini

Servings: 4
Cooking Time: 20 Minutes
Ingredients:
- 1 1/2 tablespoons butter or olive oil
- 1 minced shallot (onion or garlic works too)
- 8 ounces sliced baby Portobello mushrooms
- 1 cup cherry or grape tomatoes
- 2 cups chopped kale, stems removed
- salt to taste
- 2 avocados
- 8 pieces thick, sturdy wheat bread
- White cheese like Provolone or Mozzarella
- Olive oil

Directions:
1.   Put the butter in a big skillet and allow it to melt on medium heat. Put in the shallots and cook until they become translucent. Mix in the mushrooms, and cook until they start to brown. Then mix in the kale and tomatoes, and cook until the kale wilts, and the tomatoes are cooked through.
2.   Mash the avocados using a fork. Spread the avocado on what's going to be the inside of each piece of bread. Then place a layer of cheese on half of the pieces of bread, then a layer of veggies, and finally another layer of cheese. Top with another piece of bread. Brush the top and bottom of the sandwich with olive oil
3.   Cook the Panini on medium heat for 4 to 5 minutes, flipping halfway through. The bread should be brown, and the cheese should be melted.

29.   Peanut Butter Waffle With Banana

Servings: 1
Cooking Time: 4 Minutes
Ingredients:
- 1 Frozen Waffle
- 1 tbsp Peanut Butter
- ¼ Banana, sliced

Directions:
1.   Preheat the sandwich maker and grease it with some cooking spray.
2.   Place the waffle on top of the bottom ring.
3.   Spread the peanut butter over and close the lid.
4.   Cook for about 3 minutes.
5.   Open carefully and transfer to a plate.
6.   Top with the banana slices and enjoy!

Nutrition Info: Calories 214 Total Fats 11g Carbs 25g Protein 6.3g Fiber 2.9g

30.   Croissant Sandwich With Sausage, Egg, And Cheddar

Servings: 1
Cooking Time: 5 Minutes
Ingredients:
- 5 Slices of Cooked Sausage
- 1 Egg
- 1 slice Cheddar
- 1 Croissant
- 2 tsp Mayonnaise
- Salt and Pepper, to taste

Directions:
1. Preheat and grease the sandwich maker.
2. Cut the croissant in half and spread the mayonnaise over the cut-side of each half.
3. Place one half of the croissant with the cut-side up in the bottom ring.
4. Top with the cheddar and sausage.
5. Lower the cooking plate and crack the egg into it. Season with salt and pepper.
6. Top with the second croissant half, placing it with the cut-side down.
7. Close the unit and cook for 4 to 5 minutes.
8. Rotate clockwise carefully, and transfer to a plate.
9. Serve and enjoy!

Nutrition Info: Calories 580 Total Fats 41.5g Carbs 27g Protein 24g Fiber 1.5g

31.   Classic Egg, Ham And Cheese

Servings: 1
Cooking Time: 5 Minutes
Ingredients:
- 1 toasted English muffin, sliced
- 2 slices deli ham
- 1 slice cheddar cheese
- 1 large egg

Directions:
1. Preheat the breakfast sandwich maker.
2. Place half of the English muffin, cut-side up, inside the bottom tray of the sandwich maker.
3. Fold the slices of ham on top of the English muffin half and top with the slice of cheddar cheese.
4. Slide the egg tray into place and crack the egg into it.
5. Top the egg with the other half of the English muffin.
6. Close the sandwich maker and cook for 4 to 5 minutes until the egg is cooked through.
7. Carefully rotate the egg tray out of the sandwich maker then open the sandwich maker and enjoy your sandwich.

32.   Pita Bread Chicken Sandwich

Servings: 1
Cooking Time: 3 Minutes
Ingredients:
- 3 ounces shredded Rotisserie Chicken
- ¼ tsp Curry Powder
- 2 tsp Mayonnaise
- 1 tbsp chopped Red Pepper
- 1 tbsp chopped Celery
- 1 tbsp chopped Tomatoes
- 1 tsp chopped Parsley
- 2 small Pita Breads or one large cut into two circles that fit inside the sandwixh maker

Directions:
1. Grease the unit with cooking spray and preheat it until the green light appears.
2. Place one pita bread on top of the bottom ring.
3. Add some mayo to it and sprinkle the curry powder over.
4. Top with the chicken, veggies, ad parsley.
5. Drizzle the rest of the mayonnaise.
6. Lower the cooking plate and top ring, and then top the sandwich with the second pita bread.
7. Close and cook the sandwich for 3 minutes.
8. Rotate clockwise and lift to open.
9. Serve and enjoy!

Nutrition Info: Calories 420 Total Fats 26g Carbs 26.5g Protein 24g Fiber 3g

33.   Pulled Pork Sandwich

Servings: 1
Cooking Time: 4 Minutes
Ingredients:
- 1 smaller Hamburger Bun
- 3 ounces Pulled Pork
- 4 Red Onion Rings
- ½ Pickle, sliced
- 2 tsp Mustard

Directions:
1. Preheat the sandwich maker and grease it with some cooking spray.
2. Cut the bun in half and spread the insides with the mustard.
3. When the green light appears, place on bu half into the bottom ring with the cut-side up.
4. Top with pork, onion rings, and pickle.
5. Lower the top ring and plate and place the second bun half inside.
6. Close and cook for 4 minutes.
7. Rotate clockwise and open carefully.
8. Serve and enjoy!

Nutrition Info: Calories 372 Total Fats 18g Carbs 27g Protein 27g Fiber 2.2g

34.   Parmesan And Bacon On Whole Wheat

Servings: 1
Cooking Time: 5 Minutes
Ingredients:
- 2 slices whole wheat bread
- 3 slices bacon, cooked
- 2 tablespoons grated parmesan cheese
- 1 large egg

Directions:
1. Preheat the breakfast sandwich maker.
2. Place one piece of bread inside the bottom tray of the sandwich maker.
3. Break the pieces of bacon in half and arrange them on top of the bread.
4. Top the bacon with the grated cheese.
5. Slide the egg tray into place and crack the egg into it. Use a fork to stir the egg, just breaking the yolk.
6. Place the second piece of bread on top of the egg.
7. Close the sandwich maker and cook for 4 to 5 minutes until the egg is cooked through.
8. Carefully rotate the egg tray out of the sandwich maker then open the sandwich maker to enjoy your sandwich.

35.   Spinach And Pesto Chicken Panini

Servings: 1
Cooking Time: 5 Minutes
Ingredients:
- 1/2 cup mayonnaise
- 2 tablespoons prepared pesto
- 1 1/2 cups shredded rotisserie chicken
- Kosher salt
- Freshly ground pepper
- 1 1lb. Ciabatta loaf, split lengthwise and cut into 4 pieces
- Extra-virgin olive oil, for brushing
- 1 cup lightly packed baby spinach
- 8 thin slices of Swiss cheese

Directions:
1. Use a whisk to combine the pesto and mayonnaise. Then mix in the chicken and salt and pepper to taste.
2. Use a brush to coat the top and bottom of the bread with olive oil. Put a layer of chicken on the bottom piece of bread, then spinach, and finally cheese. Place the top piece of bread on the cheese.
3. Cook the sandwiches for 7 minutes on medium heat, and make sure to flip halfway through. The bread should be brown, and the cheese should be melted.

36.   Apple And Brie Croissant Sandwich

Servings: 1
Cooking Time: 4 Minutes
Ingredients:
- 2 Apple Slices
- 1 ounce Brie, crumbled
- 1 Croissant
- 2 tsp Cream Cheese

Directions:
1. Preheat and grease the sandwich maker.
2. Cut the croissant in half and spread one teaspoon of cream cheese over each half.
3. When the green light appears, place one of the croissant halves into the bottom ring, with the cut-side up.
4. Top with the apple slices and brie.
5. Lower the top ring and cooking plate and place the other croissant half inside.
6. Close and cook for 4 minutes.
7. Turn the handle clockwise, open, and transfer to a plate.
8. Serve and enjoy!
Nutrition Info: Calories 369 Total Fats 23g Carbs 29g Protein 11g Fiber 2g

37.   Mustardy Egg Muffin Melt

Servings: 1
Cooking Time: 4 Minutes
Ingredients:
- 1 English Muffin
- 2 ounces shredded Cheddar Cheese
- 2 tsp Yellow Mustard
- 1 Egg
- Salt and Pepper, to taste
- 1 tsp chopped Parsley

Directions:
1. Preheat and grease the sandwich maker with cooking spray.
2. Cut the English muffin in half and brush the insides with the mustard.
3. Whisk the egg and season it with salt and pepper. Stir in the chopped parsley.
4. When the green light appears, place half of the muffin in the bottom ring, with the cut-side down.
5. Top with the cheese.
6. Lower the top ring and cooking plate, and pour the whisked egg into the plate.
7. Top with the second muffin half, keeping the cut-side down.
8. Close and cook for 4 minutes.
9. Rotate clockwise and open.
10. Transfer the sandwich to a plate and enjoy!

Nutrition Info: Calories 435 Total Fats 25g Carbs 27g Protein 26g Fiber 2.3g

38.   Egg And Cheddar Cheese Biscuit

Servings: 1
Cooking Time: 5 Minutes
Ingredients:
- 1 biscuit, sliced
- 1 slice cheddar cheese
- 1 slice red onion
- 1 slice green pepper, seeded and cored
- 1 large egg

Directions:
1. Preheat the breakfast sandwich maker.
2. Place half of the biscuit, cut-side up, inside the bottom tray of the sandwich maker.
3. Top the biscuit with a slice of cheddar cheese along with the red onion and green pepper.
4. Slide the egg tray into place and crack the egg into it.
5. Top the egg with the other half of the biscuit.
6. Close the sandwich maker and cook for 4 to 5 minutes until the egg is cooked through.
7. Carefully rotate the egg tray out of the sandwich maker then open the sandwich maker and enjoy your sandwich.

39.   Ground Turkey Taco Cups

Servings: 1
Cooking Time: 5 Minutes
Ingredients:
- 1 Flour Tortilla
- 1 ounce shredded Cheddar
- 1 tsp Sour Cream
- 1 tsp Salsa
- 2 ounces cooked Ground Chicken
- 2 tsp chopped Onion
- 1 tsp chopped Parsley

Directions:
1. Preheat and grease the sandwich maker.
2. Slide out the cooking plate – you will not need it for this recipe.
3. Place the tortilla into the ring, tucking it, so that it looks like a cup.
4. In a small bowl, combine the rest of the ingredients.
5. Fill the taco cup with the chicken filling.
6. Close the lid and cook for 5 minutes.
7. Rotate clockwise and lift to open, then transfer to a plate.
8. Serve and enjoy!

Nutrition Info: Calories 305 Total Fats 14.5g Carbs 19.6g Protein 23.2g Fiber 1.3g

40.   Caramel Strawberries Sandwich

Servings: 4
Cooking Time: 5minutes
Ingredients:
- 4 Butter Croissants, large
- 4 tbsp. Caramel Sauce, salted
- 8 sliced Strawberries
- 9 Marshmallows, large, cut into slices
- Cooking spray

Directions:
1. Slice the croissants in half. Spread ½ tbsp. of caramel on each.
2. On one of the sides layer the strawberry slices and on the other layer the marshmallow slices.
3. Bring the sides together to make a sandwich.
4. Preheat the sandwich maker and spray with a cooking spray.
5. Cook the sandwiches for 2 minutes and flip. Cook for 2 more minutes
6. Remove and let it rest for 1 minutes
7. Cut in half and serve.

41.   Bruschetta Turkey Panini

Servings: 4
Cooking Time: 4 Minutes
Ingredients:
- 8 slices Italian bread
- 8 fresh basil leaves
- 8 thinly sliced tomatoes
- 16 slices of Black Pepper Turkey Breast
- 4 pieces of mozzarella cheese
- 4 tablespoons mayonnaise
- Olive oil

Directions:
1. Cut the basil into ribbons.
2. Place a layer of turkey on a piece of bread, then basil, and then cheese. Spread the mayo on the bottom part of the top piece of bread, and place it on top of the cheese. Brush the top and bottom of the sandwich with olive oil
3. Cook the sandwiches for 4 minutes on medium heat, and make sure to flip halfway through. The bread should be brown, and the cheese should be melted.

42.   Veggie Pepper Jack Sandwich With Arugula

Servings: 1
Cooking Time: 4 Minutes
Ingredients:
- 1 multigrain English muffin, split
- Sliced onion, bell pepper and radish
- A few arugula leaves
- 1 slice Pepper Jack cheese
- 1 egg

Directions:
1. Place one English muffin half, cut side up into the bottom ring of breakfast sandwich maker. Place slices of onion, bell pepper, radish, arugula leaves and Pepper Jack cheese on top.
2. Lower the cooking plate and top ring; crack an egg into the egg plate and pierce to break the yolk. Top with other muffin half.
3. Close the cover and cook for 4 to 5 minutes or until egg is cooked through. Gently slide the egg plate out and remove sandwich with a rubber spatula.

43.   Meat Lovers Sandwich

Servings: 1
Cooking Time: 5 Minutes
Ingredients:
- 2 slices flatbread
- 1 tsp. Dijon mustard
- 1 slice ham
- 2 slices bacon
- 1 precooked sausage patty
- 1 slice smoked Gouda cheese
- 1 egg
- Sea salt and pepper

Directions:
1.   Spread Dijon mustard on both flatbread slices. Place one slice into the bottom ring of breakfast sandwich maker, mustard side up. Place ham, bacon, sausage and Gouda cheese on top.
2.   Lower the cooking plate and top ring; crack an egg into the egg plate and pierce to break the yolk. Season with sea salt and pepper and top with other piece of flatbread.
3.   Close the cover and cook for 4 to 5 minutes or until egg is cooked through. Gently slide the egg plate out and remove sandwich with a rubber spatula.

44.   Peanut Butter Magic

Servings: 1
Cooking Time: 4 Minutes
Ingredients:
- 1 cinnamon and raisin bagel, split
- 1 Tbsp. peanut butter
- 2 tsp. honey
- Banana slices
- Apple slices
- Dash of cinnamon

Directions:
1.   Spread peanut butter on both bagel halves. Place one half into the bottom ring of breakfast sandwich maker, peanut butter side up. Drizzle honey and place banana and apple slices on top. Sprinkle with cinnamon.
2.   Lower cooking plate and top ring; top with other bagel half. Close the cover and cook for 3 to 4 minutes or until sandwich is warmed. Remove from sandwich maker and enjoy!

45.   Pesto Italian Bagel

Servings: 1
Cooking Time: 5 Minutes
Ingredients:
- 1 bagel, split
- 1 Tbsp. store bought pesto
- 1 slice ham
- 4 round slices pepperoni
- 1 slice tomato
- 1 slice provolone cheese
- 1 egg

Directions:
1.   Spread pesto on both halves of bagel. Place one half, pesto side up into the bottom ring of breakfast sandwich maker. Place ham, pepperoni, tomato and provolone cheese on top.
2.   Lower the cooking plate and top ring; crack an egg into the egg plate and pierce to break the yolk; top with other bagel half.
3.   Close the cover and cook for 4 to 5 minutes or until egg is cooked through. Gently slide the egg plate out and remove sandwich with a rubber spatula.

46.   Spicy Cream Cheese Raspberry Croissant

Servings: 1
Cooking Time: 3 Minutes
Ingredients:
- 1 small croissant, sliced in half
- 1 – 2 Tbsp. cream cheese
- 1 – 2 Tbsp. raspberry jam
- 1 small jalapeño, seeded and sliced in thin rings

Directions:
1.   Spread cream cheese and raspberry jam on bottom half of croissant. Place in the bottom of breakfast sandwich maker. Sprinkle with a few jalapeño rings (to taste).
2.   Lower cooking plate and top ring. Place other half of croissant on top and close the sandwich maker lid. Cook for 2 – 3 minutes or until the cream cheese is melted and sandwich is warm. Carefully remove from sandwich maker and enjoy!

47.   Tuna And Corn Muffin Sandwich

Servings: 1
Cooking Time: 3 Minutes
Ingredients:
- 1 Whole Wheat English Muffin
- 2 ounces canned Tuna, drained
- 2 tsp Mayonnaise
- 2 tsp canned Corn
- 2 tsp chopped Tomatoes

Directions:
1. Preheat and grease the unit.
2. Cut the English muffin half.
3. When the green light appears, add half of the muffin to the bottom ring.
4. Combine together the tuna, mayonnaise, tomatoes, and corn.
5. Place the tuna mixture on top of the muffin half.
6. Lower the top ring and add the second half of the muffin.
7. Close the unit and cook for 3 minutes.
8. Rotate clockwise and open. Transfer to a plate.
9. Serve and enjoy!

Nutrition Info: Calories 255 Total Fats 9g Carbs 29.5g Protein 17g Fiber 5g

48.   Banana Foster Sandwich

Servings: 8
Cooking Time: 10minutes
Ingredients:
- 4 oz. softened Cream Cheese
- 2 tbsp. of Brown sugar
- ½ cup Bananas, chopped
- 2 oz. Chocolate, chopped, Semi-Sweet
- 8 Bread slices, Italian bread
- 2 tbsp. melted butter

Directions:
1. Preheat the sandwich maker.
2. In a bowl combine the sugar and cream cheese. Blend until soft. Add the chocolate and bananas, mix again.
3. Spread on 4 Italian bread slices and cover with the other bread slices.
4. Brush sides with butter.
5. Grill for about 2 minutes.
6. Cut the sandwiches in half and serve.

49.   Chocolate Donut Dessert Sandwich

Servings: 1
Cooking Time: 5 Minutes
Ingredients:
- 1 chocolate-frosted glazed donut, sliced in half
- 2 tbsp. chocolate hazelnut spread
- 1 ounce cream cheese
- ½ cup sliced strawberries

Directions:
1. Divide the two tablespoons chocolate hazelnut spread between the donut halves, spreading it evenly along the cut edges.
2. Preheat the breakfast sandwich maker.
3. Place half of the donut inside the bottom tray of the sandwich maker.
4. Top the donut with cream cheese and strawberries.
5. Place the second half of the donut on top of the strawberries.
6. Close the sandwich maker and cook for 4 to 5 minutes until heated through.
7. Carefully open the sandwich maker and enjoy your sandwich.

50.   Creamy Brie & Fruit Sandwich

Servings: 1
Cooking Time: 5 Minutes
Ingredients:
- 2 slices crusty white bread, crusts removed
- 1 – 2 Tbsp. soft brie cheese
- 2 strawberries, sliced
- 3 – 4 grapes, sliced
- A few blueberries
- 1 Tbsp. finely chopped pecans
- Honey

Directions:
1. Spread brie cheese on both bread slices. Place one slice into the bottom ring of breakfast sandwich maker, brie side up. Place sliced strawberries, grapes, blueberries and chopped pecans on top. Drizzle with honey.
2. Lower the cooking plate and top ring; top with other slice of bread. Close the cover and cook for 3 to 4 minutes or until sandwich is warm and cheese is melted. Remove sandwich with a rubber spatula and enjoy!

51.   Hummus And Vegetable Panini

Servings: 4
Cooking Time: 5 Minutes
Ingredients:
- 1 tablespoons olive oil
- 1 small onion, sliced
- 1 medium zucchini, thinly sliced
- 1 medium cucumber, thinly sliced
- 1 red bell pepper, sliced
- 8 slices whole grain bread
- 4 tablespoon homemade or store bought hummus of your choice
- fresh spinach leaves
- 1 cup matchstick carrots
- slice of provolone cheese

Directions:
1. Spread the hummus on 1 side of 4 pieces of bread. Layer the vegetables starting with the zucchini, then, cucumber, then spinach then red bell pepper, then carrots. Top the vegetables with a slice of cheese and place another piece of bread on the cheese. Brush the top and bottom of the sandwich with the olive oil
2. Cook the Panini on medium heat for 4 to 5 minutes, flipping halfway through. The bread should be brown, and the cheese should be melted.

52.   Greek Cucumber-yogurt Flatbread

Servings: 1
Cooking Time: 5 Minutes
Ingredients:
- 2 slices flatbread
- 1 Tbsp. plain yogurt
- 1 slice tomato
- Cucumber slices
- Feta cheese
- Fresh chopped parsley
- 1 Tbsp. milk
- 1 egg
- Sea salt and pepper

Directions:
1.   Spread yogurt on both slices of flatbread. Place one slice into the bottom ring of breakfast sandwich maker, yogurt side up. Place tomato, cucumber slices, feta cheese and some fresh parsley on top.
2.   In a small bowl, whisk together milk, egg, sea salt and pepper. Lower the cooking plate and top ring; pour egg mixture into the egg plate. Top with other piece of flatbread.
3.   Close the cover and cook for 4 to 5 minutes. Slide the egg plate out and remove sandwich with a rubber spatula.

53.   Sweet And Salty Bacon Cheesy Panini

Servings: 4
Cooking Time: 3 Minutes
Ingredients:
- 8 oz. Brie, thinly sliced
- 8 pieces thick cut bacon, fully cooked
- 8 pieces Raisin-walnut bread
- ½ cup Apple butter
- Butter, softened

Directions:
1.   Spread the apple butter on one side of each piece of bread. Then add 2 pieces of bacon to apple butter side of one piece of bread and top with ¼ of the cheese. Place another piece of bread on top with the apple butter side of the bread touching the cheese. Spread butter on the other side of both pieces of bread.
2.   Cook the Panini on medium high heat for 2-3 minutes, flipping halfway through. The bread should be brown when ready.

54.   Donut Breakfast Sandwich

Servings: 1
Cooking Time: 5 Minutes
Ingredients:
- 1 glazed donut, cut in half
- 2 slices cooked bacon
- 1 slice provolone cheese
- 1 large egg

Directions:
1.   Preheat the breakfast sandwich maker.
2.   Place half of the donut, cut-side up, inside the bottom tray of the sandwich maker.
3.   Cut or break the bacon slices in half and place them on top of the donut half. Top with the slice of provolone cheese.
4.   Slide the egg tray into place and crack the egg into it.
5.   Top the egg with the other half of the donut.
6.   Close the sandwich maker and cook for 4 to 5 minutes until the egg is cooked through.
7.   Carefully rotate the egg tray out of the sandwich maker then open the sandwich maker and enjoy your sandwich.

55.   Muffin Sandwich With Egg, Ham, And Cheese

Servings: 1
Cooking Time: 5 Minutes
Ingredients:
- 1 slice Cheese
- 1 English Muffin
- 1 slice Canadian Bacon
- 1 Egg, scrambled

Directions:
1.   Preheat and grease the sandwich maker.
2.   Cut the English muffin in half and place one half with the spilt-side up into the bottom ring.
3.   Top with the bacon and cheese.
4.   Now, lower the cooking plate and add the egg inside.
5.   Close and let cook for 4-5 minutes.
6.   Slide clockwise to open using mittens.
7.   Remove the sandwich carefully and transfer to a plate.
8.   Serve and enjoy!
Nutrition Info: Calories 357 Total Fats 17g Carbs 26g Protein 24g Fiber 2g

56.   Muffuletta Breakfast Sandwich

Servings: 1
Cooking Time: 5 Minutes
Ingredients:
- 2 slices thick white bread
- 1 slice deli ham
- 1 slice hard salami
- 1 slice provolone cheese
- 1 tbsp. chopped black olives
- 1 tbsp. roasted red pepper, chopped
- 1 teaspoon minced red onion
- 1 clove garlic, minced
- Salt and pepper to taste
- 1 large egg

Directions:
1. Stir together the olives, red pepper, red onion and garlic. Season with salt and pepper and stir well.
2. Preheat the breakfast sandwich maker.
3. Place one slice of bread inside the bottom tray of the sandwich maker.
4. Layer the ham and salami over the bread and top with the olive mixture.
5. Top the olive mixture with the slice of provolone cheese.
6. Slide the egg tray into place and crack the egg into it. Stir the egg gently to break the yolk.
7. Top the egg with the other piece of bread.
8. Close the sandwich maker and cook for 4 to 5 minutes until the egg is cooked through.
9. Carefully rotate the egg tray out of the sandwich maker then open the sandwich maker and enjoy your sandwich.

57.   Blueberry Marshmallow Sandwich

Servings: 2- 4
Cooking Time: 5minutes
Ingredients:
- 4 slices of sandwich bread
- Butter, salted, at room temperature
- 6 Marshmallows, jumbo size
- ½ cup chocolate chips, white
- ½ cup Blueberries, fresh

Directions:
1. Preheat the sandwich maker.
2. Spread butter on all sides on each slice of bread.
3. Cut the marshmallow in three pieces and place them on the bread slice. Top with chocolate and then with blueberries. Cover with a bread slice.
4. Carefully place the 2 sandwiches on the sandwich maker and press hard.
5. Cook for 2 minutesutes and then flip. Cook for 2 more minutes.
6. Serve as it is or cut in half.
7. Enjoy!

58.   Biscuit Sandwich

Servings: 2 - 4
Cooking Time: 15minutes
Ingredients:
- 4 eggs
- 4 eggs, the whites
- 2 tbsp. cream
- ¼ tsp. of Garlic salt
- 6 Bacon Slices
- ¾ cup Cheddar cheese, shredded
- 4 biscuits, refrigerated

Directions:
1.   In a bowl combine the egg whites, eggs, garlic salt, and cream. Whisk well and cook them until fluffy and light.
2.   Cook the slices of bacon and then set aside. (You can prepare the first 2 steps ahead but keep them in the fridge until you are ready to prepare the sandwich.)
3.   Spray the press with cooking oil and layer with half biscuits. Top with ¼ eggs, bacon, 2 tbsp. cheese and top with the other biscuit.
4.   Cook for 5 minutes and serve.

59.   Red Pepper And Goat Cheese Sandwich

Servings: 1
Cooking Time: 5 Minutes
Ingredients:
- 2 slices multigrain bread
- 1 ounce goat cheese
- 2 slices fresh red pepper
- 1 slice red onion
- Salt and pepper to taste
- 1 large egg

Directions:
1.   Preheat the breakfast sandwich maker.
2.   Place one slice of bread inside the bottom tray of the sandwich maker.
3.   Top the bread with the goat cheese, red pepper and red onion. Season with salt and pepper to taste.
4.   Slide the egg tray into place and crack the egg into it. Use a fork to stir the egg, just breaking the yolk.
5.   Place the second slice of bread on top of the egg.
6.   Close the sandwich maker and cook for 4 to 5 minutes until the egg is cooked through.
7.   Carefully rotate the egg tray out of the sandwich maker then open the sandwich maker to enjoy your sandwich.

60.   Cheesy Beef And Egg Sandwich

Servings: 1
Cooking Time: 4 Minutes
Ingredients:
- 2 ounces cooked ground Beef
- 2 Bread Slices
- 1 Egg
- 1 ounce shredded Cheddar
- 1 tsp Mayonnaise
- Salt and Pepper, to taste

Directions:
1. Preheat the sandwich maker until the green light appears, and grease it with some cooking spray.
2. Cut the bread slices so they can fit inside the sandwich maker, and place one on top of the bottom ring.
3. Add the beef and cheddar and lower the top ring and cooking plate.
4. Crack the egg into the plate and season it with salt and pepper.
5. Brush the second slices with the mayo and place it with the mayo-side down.
6. Close the lid and cook for 4 minutes.
7. Slide out the cooking plate and open the lid carefully.
8. Tranfer to a plate with a spatula that is not metal.
9. Serve and enjoy!

Nutrition Info: Calories 590 Total Fats 35g Carbs 38g Protein 31g Fiber 6g

61.   Harissa Avocado Sausage And Egg Breakfast Panini

Servings: 2
Cooking Time: 6 Minutes
Ingredients:
- 4 pieces of sourdough or crusty bread
- ¼ cup Harissa
- 2 eggs
- ½ avocado, sliced into pieces
- 1 cup pepper jack cheese
- A handful of arugula
- 2 Merguez sausages, cooked
- Olive oil
- 2 teaspoon butter

Directions:
1. Use a whisk to beat the egg with a pinch of salt and pepper. Place the butter in a skillet and melt it on medium heat. Use a spoon to stir the eggs and push them across the pan. Cook until the eggs set, about 1 to 2 minutes.
2. Chop the sausage into small pieces or butterfly them. Spread the Harissa on what's going to be the inside of two pieces of bread. Put a layer of egg on the Harissa side of the 2 pieces of bread, then the sausage, then the arugula, then avocado and top with the cheese. Then place the other two pieces of bread on top of the cheese. Brush the top and bottom of the sandwiches with olive oil.
3. Cook the Panini on medium heat for 4 to 6 minutes, flipping halfway through. The bread should be toasted, and the cheese should be melted.

62.   Egg Whites With Mozzarella

Servings: 1
Cooking Time: 5 Minutes
Ingredients:
- 1 thin sandwich bun, sliced
- 1 thick slice tomato
- 1 slice mozzarella cheese
- 2 large egg whites, beaten

Directions:
1. Preheat the breakfast sandwich maker.
2. Place half of the sandwich bun, cut-side up, inside the bottom tray of the sandwich maker.
3. Arrange the slices of tomato and mozzarella cheese over the sandwich bun.
4. Slide the egg tray into place and crack the egg into it.
5. Top the egg with the other half of the sandwich bun.
6. Close the sandwich maker and cook for 4 to 5 minutes until the egg is cooked through.
7. Carefully rotate the egg tray out of the sandwich maker then open the sandwich maker and enjoy your sandwich.

63.   Chocolate Chip Waffle Sandwich

Servings: 1
Cooking Time: 5 Minutes
Ingredients:
- 2 small frozen waffles
- 1 Tbsp. cream cheese
- 1 Tbsp. mini chocolate chips
- 1 Tbsp. milk
- 1 egg
- Sea salt and pepper

Directions:
1. Spread cream cheese on both waffles. Place one, cream cheese side up into the bottom ring of breakfast sandwich maker. Place chocolate chips on top.
2. In a small bowl, whisk together milk, egg, sea salt and pepper. Lower the cooking plate and top ring; pour egg mixture into egg plate. Top with other waffle.
3. Close the cover and cook for 4 to 5 minutes or until egg is cooked through. Gently slide the egg plate out, remove sandwich with a rubber spatula and enjoy!

64.   Ricotta Basil Biscuit With Nectarines

Servings: 1
Cooking Time: 5 Minutes
Ingredients:
- 1 buttermilk biscuit, sliced
- 1 ripe nectarine, peeled and sliced
- 1 tbsp. ricotta cheese
- 1 tbsp. maple syrup
- 2 tsp. brown sugar

Directions:
1. Place the nectarines in a bowl and add the ricotta, maple syrup and brown sugar then toss well.
2. Preheat the breakfast sandwich maker.
3. Place half of the biscuit, cut-side up, inside the bottom tray of the sandwich maker.
4. Top the muffin with the nectarine slices, ricotta, maple syrup and brown sugar mixture
5. Place the second half of the biscuit on top of the nectarines.
6. Close the sandwich maker and cook for 4 to 5 minutes until heated through.
7. Carefully open the sandwich maker and enjoy your sandwich.

65.   Prosciutto And Fig Panini

Servings: 4
Cooking Time: 6 Minutes
Ingredients:
- 8 (0.9-ounce) slices crusty Chicago-style Italian bread
- 4 ounces very thinly sliced prosciutto
- 1 1/4 cups (4 ounces) shredded Fontina cheese
- 1/2 cup baby arugula leaves
- 1/4 cup fig preserves
- Olive oil

Directions:
1. Lightly coat the one side of each piece of bread with olive oil using a brush.
2. Spread the fig preserve on 4 pieces of bread (not on the olive oil side). On the other pieces of bread put a layer of prosciutto, then arugula and top with cheese. Place the fig coated bread on top with the fig side touching the cheese.
3. Cook the Panini on medium heat for 6 minutes, flipping halfway through. The bread should be brown, and the cheese should be melted.

66.   Nutella Sandwich

Servings: 1
Cooking Time: 5minutes
Ingredients:
- 1 tbsp. Nutella
- 2 slices of French bread
- 1 tbsp. Marshmallow Cream
- ½ Banana, sliced
- Butter

Directions:
1. Heat the sandwich maker.
2. Spread Nutella on one side of the bread slice and the marshmallow crema on another. Place the banana slices on the marshmallow cream and sandwich both sides together. Batter the outside.
3. Press with the sandwich maker and cook for about 5 minutes.
4. Serve and enjoy!

67.   Avocado, Swiss And Bacon

Servings: 1
Cooking Time: 5 Minutes
Ingredients:
- 1 croissant, sliced
- 2 slices bacon, cooked
- 1 slice Swiss cheese
- ¼ avocado, pitted and sliced
- 1 large egg
- 1 tablespoon basil pesto

Directions:
1. Divide the pesto between the two halves of the croissant, spreading it evenly.
2. Preheat the breakfast sandwich maker.
3. Place half of the croissant, pesto-side up, inside the bottom tray of the sandwich maker.
4. Arrange the slices of bacon on top of the bagel and top with the slice of Swiss cheese.
5. Slide the egg tray into place and crack the egg into it.
6. Top the egg with the other half of the croissant, pesto-side down.
7. Close the sandwich maker and cook for 4 to 5 minutes until the egg is cooked through.
8. Carefully rotate the egg tray out of the sandwich maker then open the sandwich maker and enjoy your sandwich.

68.   Salsa And Shrimp Biscuit Sandwich

Servings: 1
Cooking Time: 3 Minutes
Ingredients:
- 4 small Shrimp, cooked
- ½ tbsp Salsa
- 2 tsp Cream Cheese
- 1 ounce shredded Mozzarella Cheese
- 1 Biscuit

Directions:
1. Preheat the sandwich maker and grease it with some cooking spray.
2. Cut the biscuit in half and spread the cream cheese over the insides.
3. Add one half of the biscuit to the bottom ring, with the cream cheese up.
4. Top with the shrimp and salsa, and sprinkle the mozzarella cheese over.
5. Lower the top ring and add the second biscuit half, with the cream cheese down.
6. Close the unit and cook for 3 minutes.
7. Rotate clockwise and open carefully.
8. Serve and enjoy!

Nutrition Info: Calories 222 Total Fats 11g Carbs 13g Protein 19g Fiber 0.5g

69.   Choco-coconut Nut Quesadilla

Servings: 1
Cooking Time: 3 Minutes
Ingredients:
- 2 small corn tortillas
- 2 tsp. chocolate hazelnut spread
- 2 tsp. almond butter
- Shredded coconut
- Honey or agave nectar
- Cinnamon

Directions:
1. Spread chocolate hazelnut spread and almond butter on both tortillas. Place one tortilla into the bottom ring of breakfast sandwich maker, nut butter side up. Sprinkle with coconut, drizzle with honey or agave and add a dash of cinnamon. Cover with other tortilla
2. Close the cover and cook for 3 to 4 minutes or until warmed through. Gently remove with a rubber spatula. Slice in half or roll up.

70.   Chocolate Banana Croissant

Servings: 1
Cooking Time: 3 Minutes
Ingredients:
- 1 small croissant, sliced in half
- 1 Tbsp. chocolate hazelnut spread
- 3 – 4 slices of banana
- Shredded coconut

Directions:
1. Spread chocolate hazelnut spread on bottom half of croissant. Place in the bottom of breakfast sandwich maker. Place banana slices on top. Sprinkle with some shredded coconut.
2. Lower cooking plate and top ring. Place other half of croissant on top and close the sandwich maker lid. Cook for 2 – 3 minutes or until the croissant is warmed through. Carefully remove from sandwich maker. Enjoy immediately.

71. Buffalo Patty Melt Panini

Servings: 4
Cooking Time: 4 Minutes
Ingredients:
- 2 tablespoons unsalted butter
- 1 large Vidalia or other sweet onion, sliced
- 1 pound lean ground beef
- 1 tablespoon Worcestershire sauce
- 1/2 teaspoon garlic powder
- 1/4 teaspoon black pepper
- 8 slices seedless rye
- 1/4 pound thinly sliced Swiss cheese, about 8 slices
- 1/4 cup blue cheese dressing
- 1 cup mayonnaise
- 1 cup buffalo hot sauce

Directions:
1. Melt the butter in a large skillet on medium heat. Add the onions and cook for about 20 minutes. While the onions are cooking combine the beef, Worcestershire sauce, and the seasoning. Form the beef into patties that are similar in shape to the bread. Place the patties in the skillet with the onions for the last 5 minutes of cooking. Flip the meat once halfway through.
2. Mix the buffalo sauce and mayonnaise in a medium bowl.
3. Spread the buffalo sauce mixture on one side of each piece of bread.
4. Put a slice of cheese on a piece of bread then a patty, the onions and top with another slice of cheese and top with another piece of bread. Repeat the process with the remaining sandwiches.
5. Cook the sandwiches for 4 minutes on medium heat, and make sure to flip halfway through. The bread should be brown, and the cheese should be melted. Serve the sandwiches with a side of the blue cheese dressing.

72. Peanut Butter Bagel Sandwich

Servings: 4
Cooking Time: 5minutes
Ingredients:
- 4 Bagels, split
- ½ cup Marshmallows, minutesi
- ¼ cup chunks milk Chocolate
- ¼ cup Peanut butter, creamy
- 4 tbsp. unsalted Butter

Directions:
1. Preheat the sandwich maker on medium heat.
2. On one half spread the peanut butter evenly. Top with marshmallows and chocolate chunks. Top with the other half of the beagles.
3. Butter the sandwich maker and add the sandwiches. Press and cook for 5 minutesutes, or until the marshmallows and chocolate melt.
4. Let it cool for about 10 minutes.
5. Serve and enjoy!

73.   Chocolate Hazelnut Croissant With Blueberries And Raspberries

Servings: 1
Cooking Time: 4 Minutes
Ingredients:
- 1 small croissant, sliced in half
- 1 Tbsp. chocolate hazelnut spread
- 1 Tbsp. crushed hazelnuts
- A few fresh blueberries and raspberries

Directions:
1.   Spread chocolate hazelnut spread on bottom half of croissant. Place in the bottom of breakfast sandwich maker. Sprinkle with hazelnuts and berries.
2.   Lower the cooking plate and top ring. Place other half of croissant on top and close the sandwich maker lid. Cook for 2 – 3 minutes or until croissant is warm. Carefully remove from sandwich maker and enjoy!

74.   Beef And Veggies Bagel Sandwich

Servings: 1
Cooking Time: 3 Minutes
Ingredients:
- 1 tsp canned Peas
- 1 tsp canned Corn
- 1 tsp chopped Celery
- 1 tsp chopped Onion
- 1 Tomato Slice, chopped
- 2 ounces cooked Beef Roast, chopped
- 1 tbsp Sandwich Sauce
- 1 tbsp Cream Cheese
- 1 Bagel

Directions:
1.   Preheat the sandwich maker and grease it with some cooking spray.
2.   Cut the bagel in half and spread the cream cheese over.
3.   Place one half of the bagel on top of the bottom ring, with the spread-side up.
4.   Top with the beef and veggies, and drizzle the sauce over.
5.   Lower the top ring and add the second bagel half inside, with the cream cheese down.
6.   Close the lid and cook for 3 minutes.
7.   Rotate clockwise and open carefully.
8.   Serve and enjoy!
Nutrition Info: Calories 420 Total Fats 25g Carbs 28g Protein 23g Fiber 5g

75.   Spinach Havarti Sandwich

Servings: 1
Cooking Time: 4 Minutes
Ingredients:
- 1 English muffin
- 2 tsp. mayonnaise
- ½ tsp. yellow mustard
- A few baby spinach leaves
- 1 slice Havarti cheese
- 1 egg
- Sea salt and pepper

Directions:
1.   Spread the mayonnaise and mustard on both halves of English muffin. Place one half, mayo/mustard side up into the bottom ring of breakfast sandwich maker. Place baby spinach leaves and Havarti cheese on top.
2.   Lower the cooking plate and top ring; crack an egg into the egg plate and pierce to break the yolk. Sprinkle some sea salt and pepper on the egg and top with other muffin half.
3.   Close the cover and cook for 4 to 5 minutes or until egg is cooked through. Gently slide the egg plate out and remove sandwich with a rubber spatula.

76.   Bacon Cheddar And Tomato Panini

Servings: 4
Cooking Time: 7 Minutes
Ingredients:
- 4 Roma tomatoes, halved lengthwise, pulp and seeds removed
- olive oil
- coarse sea salt
- fresh ground black pepper
- 8 basil leaves, thinly sliced
- 2 tablespoons unsalted butter, melted
- 8 slices sourdough bread
- 8 slices bacon, fully cooked
- 4 ounces sharp cheddar cheese, thinly sliced

Directions:
1.   Preheat a small skillet on high heat.
2.   Use a brush to coat the cut side of the tomatoes with olive oil and salt and pepper to taste. Put the tomatoes on the skillet with the cut side down. Allow them to cook for 10 to 12 minutes. The tomatoes. Flip the tomatoes about halfway through. The tomatoes should be wrinkly and the tomatoes should be soft to the touch. Check the tomatoes constantly throughout the process so they don't overcook. Once cooked take them out of the skillet and season with basil.
3.   Spread the butter on one side of each piece of bread. Place 2 pieces of bacon on the unbuttered side of a piece of bread, then 2 tomatoes and a ¼ of the cheese. Then top with the other piece of bread making sure the butter side is on top.
4.   Cook the Panini on medium heat for 5-7 minutes, flipping halfway through. The bread should be brown, and the cheese should be melted.

77.   Smoked Provolone And Turkey Panini

Servings: 4
Cooking Time: 10 Minutes
Ingredients:
- 1 round Asiago Cheese Focaccia
- 3 tablespoons light mayonnaise
- 2 teaspoons Dijon mustard
- 5 ounces thinly sliced smoked provolone
- 8 ounces thinly sliced smoked turkey breast
- 1 ripe beefsteak tomato, thinly sliced
- 1 ounce baby spinach leaves
- Olive oil

Directions:
1.   Cut the bread in half horizontally.
2.   Spread a layer of mayonnaise and a layer of mustard on the inside of the top piece of bread. Place a layer of turkey on the inside of the bottom piece of bread then, spinach, then tomatoes, and top with cheese. Place the top piece of bread on the cheese with the mayonnaise side down. If necessary cut the sandwiches into wedges in order to fit it in your flip sandwich maker.
3.   Cook the sandwiches for 6 to 10 minutes on medium heat, and make sure to flip halfway through. The bread should be toasted, and the cheese should be melted. Cut the sandwiches into 4 wedges if you haven't already done so.

78.   Cheddar Hash Brown Biscuit

Servings: 1
Cooking Time: 5 Minutes
Ingredients:
- 1 buttermilk biscuit, sliced
- 1 frozen hash brown patty
- 1 slice cheddar cheese
- 1 large egg

Directions:
1.   Heat the butter in a small skillet over medium heat. Add the hash brown patty and cook for 2 to 3 minutes until lightly browned on the underside.
2.   Flip the patty and cook until browned on the other side. Remove from heat.
3.   Preheat the breakfast sandwich maker.
4.   Place half of the biscuit, cut-side up, inside the bottom tray of the sandwich maker.
5.   Top the biscuit with the cooked hash brown patty and cheddar cheese slice.
6.   Slide the egg tray into place and crack the egg into it. Use a fork to stir the egg, just breaking the yolk.
7.   Place the second half of the biscuit on top of the egg.
8.   Close the sandwich maker and cook for 4 to 5 minutes until the egg is cooked through.
9.   Carefully rotate the egg tray out of the sandwich maker then open the sandwich maker to enjoy your sandwich.

79.   Pork And Egg Tortilla Open Sandwich

Servings: 1
Cooking Time: 4 Minutes
Ingredients:
- 1 Wheat Tortilla
- 1 Egg
- 2 ounces cooked ground Pork
- 1 ounce shredded Cheddar Cheese
- 1 tbsp chopped Red Onion
- 1 tbsp Salsa

Directions:
1. Preheat and grease the sandwich maker.
2. Cut the tortilla, if needed, to fit inside the sandwich maker, and then add it to the bottom ring.
3. Place the pork on top of it, sprinkle the cheddar over, and top with the onion.
4. Lower the top ring and crack the egg into it.
5. Close the unit and wait for about 4 minutes before rotating the handle clockwise.
6. Open and transfer to a plate carefully.
7. Top with the salsa.
8. Enjoy!

Nutrition Info: Calories 466 Total Fats 28.3g Carbs 20.5g Protein 31g Fiber 1.5g

80.   Spinach, Parmesan And Egg White

Servings: 1
Cooking Time: 5 Minutes
Ingredients:
- 1 toasted English muffin, sliced
- ½ cup baby spinach leaves
- 2 large egg whites
- 1 tablespoon grated parmesan cheese
- 1 clove garlic, minced

Directions:
1. Preheat the breakfast sandwich maker.
2. Place half of the English muffin, cut-side up, inside the bottom tray of the sandwich maker.
3. Arrange the baby spinach leaves on top of the English muffin.
4. Beat the egg whites, parmesan cheese and garlic in a small bowl.
5. Slide the egg tray into place and pour the egg mixture into it.
6. Top the egg with the other half of the English muffin.
7. Close the sandwich maker and cook for 4 to 5 minutes until the egg is cooked through.
8. Carefully rotate the egg tray out of the sandwich maker then open the sandwich maker and enjoy your sandwich.

81. Easy Bread Pudding Sandwich

Servings: 1
Cooking Time: 5 Minutes
Ingredients:
- 2 slices stale bread, cubed
- 1 large egg
- 2 tbsp. maple syrup or honey
- 2 tbsp. plain yogurt
- 1 tbsp. melted butter
- Pinch ground nutmeg
- 1 chicken sausage patty, cooked
- 1 slice Swiss cheese
- 1 large egg

Directions:
1. Arrange the chunks of bread in a small round ramekin.
2. Whisk together the remaining ingredients and pour over the bread – do not stir.
3. Microwave the ramekin on high heat for 2 minutes until the pudding is firm and hot. Let cool for 5 minutes.
4. Preheat the breakfast sandwich maker.
5. Turn the bread pudding out of the ramekin and into the bottom of the breakfast sandwich maker.
6. Top the bread pudding with the sausage patty and slice of Swiss cheese.
7. Slide the egg tray into place and crack the egg into it. Use a fork to stir the egg, just breaking the yolk.
8. Close the sandwich maker and cook for 4 to 5 minutes until the egg is cooked through.
9. Carefully rotate the egg tray out of the sandwich maker then open the sandwich maker to enjoy your sandwich.

82. Hot Pork Sausage And Srambled Egg Sandwich

Servings: 1
Cooking Time: 4 Minutes
Ingredients:
- 2 ounces ground Pork Sausage, cooked
- 1 ounce shredded Cheddar Cheese
- 1 Egg
- ¼ tsp dried Thyme
- 1 Biscuit
- ½ tsp Hot Pepper Sauce
- Salt and Pepper, to taste

Directions:
1. Preheat and grease the sandwich maker with cooking spray.
2. Cut the biscuit in half and place one half inside the bottom ring.
3. Top with the sausage and cheddar, and sprinkle the hot sauce over.
4. Lower the top ring and cooking plate, and crack the egg into it.
5. Season with salt and pepper and sprinkle the thyme over.
6. Close the unit and wait 4 minutes before rotating clockwise to open.
7. Serve and enjoy!
Nutrition Info: Calories 455 Total Fats 33g Carbs 13g Protein 26g Fiber 0.4g

83.   Cheesy Chicken Waffle Sandwich

Servings: 1
Cooking Time: 4 ½ Minutes
Ingredients:
- A couple of thin cooked Chicken Slices, about 2-3 ounces in total
- 1 slice American or Cheddar Cheese
- 1 Prosciutto Slice
- 2 tomato Slices
- 2 tsp Mayonnaise
- 2 Frozen Waffles

Directions:
1. Preheat and grease the sandwich maker.
2. Cut the waffles into 4-inch circles so that they can fit inside the unit.
3. Place on waffle on top of the bottom ring.
4. Add the chicken, place the tomato sliced on top, and spread the mayo over.
5. Top with the prosciutto and finish it off by adding the slice of cheese.
6. Lower the top ring and add the second waffle.
7. Close the unit and cook for 4 ½ minutes.
8. Serve and enjoy!

Nutrition Info: Calories 350 Total Fats 28g Carbs 22g Protein 24g Fiber 2g

84.   Hash Browns & Sausage Sandwich

Servings: 1
Cooking Time: 10 Minutes
Ingredients:
- 2 slices multigrain bread
- 1 Tbsp. butter
- 1 cup frozen hash browns
- 1 precooked sausage patty
- 1 slice provolone cheese
- 1 egg

Directions:
1. In a small skillet heat the butter over medium heat. Place hash browns over the butter in a single layer and let fry for about 5 minutes or until a brown crust forms on the bottom.
2. Place one slice of bread into the bottom ring of breakfast sandwich maker. Top with hash browns, sausage and provolone cheese.
3. Lower the cooking plate and top ring; crack an egg into the egg plate and pierce to break the yolk. Top with other slice of bread.
4. Close the cover and cook for 4 to 5 minutes or until egg is cooked. Slide the egg plate out, remove sandwich with a rubber spatula and enjoy!

85.   Pizza Snack

Servings: 1
Cooking Time: 4 Minutes
Ingredients:
- ½ English Muffin
- 4 mini Pepeproni Slices
- 1 tbsp shredded Cheddar Cheese
- 1 tsp Ketchup

Directions:
1. Preheat the unit until the green light appears and grease it with cooking spray.
2. Add the muffin to the bottom ring.
3. Spread the ketchup over it and top with the pepperoni and cheese.
4. Close the lid and cook for 3 minutes.
5. Open carefully and transfer to a plate with a non-metal spatula.
6. Serve and enjoy!

Nutrition Info: Calories 197 Total Fats 11.7g Carbs 14g Protein 8.5g Fiber 1g

86.   Caribbean Sandwich

Servings: 1
Cooking Time: 5minutes
Ingredients:
- 2 slices of bread
- 1 tbsp. Yellow mustard
- Hot sauce to taste
- 3 slices queso Blanco
- 3 slices deli ham
- Fried or sautéed plantains
- Charred onion, red

Directions:
1. Spread the mustard on one bread slice.
2. Layer the remaining ingredients.
3. Add more queso Blanco to taste.
4. Place the second bread slice on top.
5. Press with the sandwich maker and cook for 5 minutes.
6. Serve and enjoy!

87. Raspberry Sandwich

Servings: 1
Cooking Time: 4minutes
Ingredients:
- 2 slices of Challah bread
- 2 tbsp. of Cream cheese
- ½ tbsp. Butter, melted
- 1 – 2 tbsp. Raspberry Preserves

Directions:
1. Turn on medium-high heat and preheat the sandwich maker.
2. Spread the cheese on one of the bread slices.
3. Spread the raspberry on the other bread slices.
4. Sandwich together and brush with butter.
5. Cook for 4 minutes.
6. Cut the sandwich in half and serve.

88. Muffuletta Panini

Servings: 4
Cooking Time: 4 Minutes
Ingredients:
- softened butter
- 8 slices rustic bread or 8 slices sourdough bread
- 16 slices provolone cheese (thin slices) or 16 slices mozzarella cheese (thin slices)
- 1/2 cup olive salad, drained or 1/2 cup olive tapenade
- 6 ounces thinly sliced black forest ham
- 6 ounces sliced mortadella
- 4 ounces sliced genoa salami

Directions:
1. Spread butter on both sides of each piece of bread.
2. Place 2 pieces of cheese on 4 piece of bread. Then put down a layer of olive salad, ham, mortadella, salami and top with the remaining cheese. Then top with the another piece of bread
3. Cook the Panini on medium heat for 4 minutes, flipping halfway through. The bread should be brown, and the cheese should be melted.

89.   Gluten-free Crispy Grilled Cheese And Bacon Sandwich

Servings: 1
Cooking Time: 3 ½ Minutes
Ingredients:
- 1 ounce Bacon, chopped
- 1 ounce shredded Cheddar
- 1 ounce shredded Gouda
- 2 tsp Butter
- 2 Gluten-Free Bread

Directions:
1. Preheat the unit until the green light appears. Grease with some cooking spray.
2. Spread the butter over the bread slices, and cut them to make them fit inside the unit.
3. Place one bread slice on top of the bottom ring, with the butter-side down.
4. Top with the cheese and bacon.
5. Lower the top rin and add the second slice of bread, with the butter-side up.
6. Close the lid and cook for 3 ½ minutes.
7. Rotate clockwise, open, and transfer to a plate.
8. Serve and enjoy!

Nutrition Info: Calories 430 Total Fats 22g Carbs 39g Protein 20g Fiber 5g

90.   Spicy Soppressata Panini With Pesto And Mozzarella

Servings: 4
Cooking Time: 10 Minutes
Ingredients:
- 1 Ciabatta loaf, cut into 4 portions, or 4 Ciabatta rolls
- 1/2 cup basil pesto, purchased or homemade
- 8 ounces fresh mozzarella cheese, sliced
- 4 ounces sliced spicy Soppressata salami

Directions:
1. Cut the Ciabatta in half horizontally.
2. Spread the pesto on the inside of each piece of bread. Place a layer of salami on the bottom piece of bread and then place the cheese on top. Top with the other piece of bread
3. Cook the Panini on medium high heat for 5 to 7 minutes, flipping halfway through. The bread should be brown, and the cheese should be melted.

91.   Piña Colada Croissant

Servings: 1
Cooking Time: 4 Minutes
Ingredients:
- 1 small croissant, sliced in half
- 1 Tbsp. cream cheese
- 1 – 2 Tbsp. finely chopped pineapple
- Shredded coconut
- Honey

Directions:
1. Spread cream cheese on both croissant halves. Place one half into the bottom ring of breakfast sandwich maker, cut side up. Place chopped pineapple and shredded coconut on top. Drizzle with honey.
2. Lower the cooking plate and top ring; top with other croissant half. Close the cover and cook for 3 to 4 minutes or until sandwich is warmed through. Open sandwich maker and remove sandwich.

92.   Pizza Sandwich

Servings: 1
Cooking Time: 5minutes
Ingredients:
- 2 Bread slices, sourdough
- Butter
- 4 -5 Chicken strips (you can use pre-cooked)
- 1 tbsp. Marinara sauce
- 8 slices Pepperoni
- 2 slices Cheese, Mozzarella
- ½ tbsp. Parmesan cheese, grated

Directions:
1.   Preheat the sandwich maker.
2.   Spread butter on each bread slices.
3.   On the side without butter layer the Ingredients: mozzarella, pepperoni, marinara sauce, chicken strips, and Parmesan.
4.   Top with a slice of bread but place the butter side up.
5.   Cook on the sandwich maker for about 5 minutes.
6.   Serve and enjoy!

93.   Caramel Cashew Waffle Sandwich

Servings: 1
Cooking Time: 3 Minutes
Ingredients:
- 2 small round waffles (store bought or homemade)
- 1 Tbsp. store bought caramel sauce
- 2 Tbsp. finely chopped cashews
- 2 strips bacon
- 1 egg

Directions:
1.   Spread caramel sauce on both waffles. Place one waffle into the bottom ring of breakfast sandwich maker, caramel side up. Sprinkle cashews on top, then top with bacon.
2.   Lower the cooking plate and top ring; crack an egg into the egg plate and pierce to break the yolk. Top with other waffle.
3.   Close the cover and cook for 4 to 5 minutes or until egg is cooked through. Gently slide the egg plate out and remove sandwich with a rubber spatula and slice in half.

94.   Sausage & Gravy Biscuit

Servings: 1
Cooking Time: 4 Minutes
Ingredients:
- 1 store bought or homemade biscuit, sliced in half
- 1 – 2 Tbsp. store bought country gravy
- 1 precooked sausage patty
- 1 slice cheddar cheese
- 1 egg

Directions:
1.   Spread the country gravy on both biscuit halves. Place one biscuit half, cut side up into the bottom ring of breakfast sandwich maker. Place sausage patty and cheddar cheese on top.
2.   Lower the cooking plate and top ring; crack an egg into the egg plate and pierce to break the yolk. Top with other biscuit half.
3.   Close the cover and cook for 4 to 5 minutes or until egg is cooked through. Gently slide the egg plate out and remove sandwich with a rubber spatula.

95.   Waffle, Egg And Sausage

Servings: 1
Cooking Time: 5 Minutes
Ingredients:
- 2 round frozen waffles
- 1 pork sausage patty, cooked
- 1 large egg
- 1 teaspoon maple syrup

Directions:
1.   Preheat the breakfast sandwich maker.
2.   Place one of the waffles inside the bottom tray of the sandwich maker.
3.   Put the sausage patty on top of the waffle.
4.   Slide the egg tray into place and crack the egg into it.
5.   Top the egg with the other waffle.
6.   Close the sandwich maker and cook for 4 to 5 minutes until the egg is cooked through.
7.   Carefully rotate the egg tray out of the sandwich maker then open the sandwich maker.
8.   Remove the top waffle and drizzle the egg with maple syrup.
9.   Replace the waffle and enjoy your sandwich.

96. Ultimate Blt Melt

Servings: 1
Cooking Time: 8 Minutes
Ingredients:
- 1 multigrain English muffin, split
- 1 Tbsp. mayonnaise
- 1 slice tomato
- 2 slices smoked bacon
- ½ slice cheddar cheese
- ½ slice Monterey Jack cheese
- Baby spinach leaves
- 1 Tbsp. milk
- 1 egg
- 1 Tbsp. diced onion
- 1 tsp. diced jalapeño
- Sea salt and pepper

Directions:
1. Spread mayonnaise on both English muffin halves. Place one half into the bottom ring of breakfast sandwich maker, mayo side up. Place tomato, bacon, cheddar cheese, Monterey Jack cheese and spinach leaves on top.
2. In a small bowl, whisk together milk, egg, onion, jalapeño, sea salt and pepper. Lower the cooking plate and top ring; pour in egg mixture. Top with other muffin half.
3. Close the cover and cook for 4 to 5 minutes or until egg is cooked through and cheeses are melted. Gently slide the egg plate out and remove sandwich with a rubber spatula.

97. Smoked Salmon And Brie Sandwich

Servings: 1
Cooking Time: 5 Minutes
Ingredients:
- 1 whole wheat English muffin, sliced
- 2 ounces smoked salmon
- 1 ounce Brie cheese, chopped
- 1 tbsp. chopped chives
- ½ tsp. chopped capers
- 1 large egg

Directions:
1. Preheat the breakfast sandwich maker.
2. Place half of the English muffin, cut-side up, inside the bottom tray of the sandwich maker.
3. Top the muffin with the salmon, chopped brie, chives and capers.
4. Slide the egg tray into place and crack the egg into it. Use a fork to stir the egg, just breaking the yolk.
5. Place the second half of the English muffin on top of the egg. Close the sandwich maker and cook for 4 to 5 minutes until the egg is cooked through
6. .Carefully rotate the egg tray out of the sandwich maker then open the sandwich maker to enjoy your sandwich

98.   Portabella Mushroom Sandwich

Servings: 1
Cooking Time: 5 Minutes
Ingredients:
- 1 whole wheat English muffin, sliced
- 1 teaspoon olive oil
- 1 portabella mushroom cap
- 1 slice provolone cheese
- 1 large egg
- ½ cup spring greens

Directions:
1. Brush the English muffin with olive oil.
2. Preheat the breakfast sandwich maker.
3. Place half of the English muffin, cut-side up, inside the bottom tray of the sandwich maker.
4. Put the mushroom cap on top of the English muffin.
5. Top the mushroom cap with the slice of provolone cheese.
6. Slide the egg tray into place and crack the egg into it.
7. Top the egg with the other half of the English muffin.
8. Close the sandwich maker and cook for 4 to 5 minutes until the egg is cooked through.
9. Carefully rotate the egg tray out of the sandwich maker then open the sandwich maker.
10. Remove the top English muffin half and top the sandwich with the spring greens.
11. Replace the English muffin on top and enjoy your sandwich.

99.   Maple Bacon Waffle Sandwich

Servings: 1
Cooking Time: 4 Minutes
Ingredients:
- 2 small round waffles (store bought or homemade)
- Maple syrup
- 2 strips maple bacon
- 1 slice cheddar cheese
- 1 egg
- 1 Tbsp. milk
- Sea salt and pepper

Directions:
1. Place one waffle in the bottom of sandwich maker. Drizzle some maple syrup on top, then the maple bacon and cheddar cheese.
2. Lower the cooking plate and top ring. In a small bowl, whisk together egg, milk, sea salt and pepper; pour into egg plate. Top with other waffle.
3. Close the cover and cook for 4 to 5 minutes or until egg is cooked through and cheese is melted. Slide the egg plate out and remove sandwich with a rubber spatula. Cut in half.

100. Bacon Egg And Sausage Breakfast Panini

Servings: 2
Cooking Time: 6 Minutes
Ingredients:
- 2 pita breads
- 1/2cup pesto
- 2 eggs
- 1 cup shredded sharp cheddar cheese
- 1 cup shredded Monterey Jack cheese
- 1 cup shredded mozzarella cheese
- 1 pork sausage patty, cooked
- 2 strips bacon, cooked
- 1/3 cup roasted red pepper
- 1-2 tablespoons butter, melted
- 2 scallions, chopped

Directions:
1.   Use a whisk to beat the egg with a pinch of salt and pepper. Place the butter in a skillet and melt it on medium heat. Use a spoon to stir the eggs and push them across the pan. Cook until the eggs set, about 1 to 2 minutes.
2.   Chop the sausage into small pieces. Spread the pesto on half of both pieces of pita. Top the pitas with half the cheese, then eggs, bacon, sausage, bell pepper, the remaining, cheese and then top with the scallions. Fold the other side of the pita on top of the filling, and spread the butter on the outside of the pitas.
3.   Cook the Panini on medium heat for 4 to 6 minutes, flipping halfway through. The bread should be brown, and the cheese should be melted.

101. Apple, Turkey And Cheddar Sandwich

Servings: 2
Cooking Time: 5minutes
Ingredients:
- 4 slices of Bread
- 4 tbsp. Butter
- 2 tbsp. Mustard
- 1 Apple, sliced thinly (green)
- 8 slices of Cheddar cheese, sharp
- 8 slices of deli turkey, roasted

Directions:
1.   Preheat the sandwich press.
2.   Spread 1 tbsp. butter on each bread slice.
3.   Spread mustard on 2 bread slices. Lay the turkey, cheese and apple slices. Top with on bread slice.
4.   Grill for about 5 minutes.
5.   Let it rest for 1 minutes and serve.

102.   Pancake, Sausage & Egg Sandwich

Servings: 1
Cooking Time: 3 Minutes
Ingredients:
- 2 small store bought or homemade pancakes
- Butter
- 1 sausage patty
- 1 slice cheddar cheese
- 1 egg

Directions:
1.   Butter each pancake and place one, butter side up, into the bottom ring of breakfast sandwich maker. Place sausage patty and cheddar cheese on top.
2.   Lower the cooking plate and top ring; crack an egg into the egg plate and pierce to break the yolk; top with other buttered pancake.
3.   Close the cover and cook for 4 to 5 minutes or until egg is cooked through. Gently slide the egg plate out and remove sandwich with a rubber spatula.

103.   Quick And Easy Quesadillas

Servings: 1
Cooking Time: 5 Minutes
Ingredients:
- 2 small round tortillas
- 2 slices cooked bacon
- 1 ounce shredded cheddar jack cheese
- 1 tbsp. minced red onion
- 1 tbsp. minced red pepper
- 1 tbsp. BBQ sauce
- 1 large egg
- 1 tbsp. fresh salsa
- 1 tbsp. sour cream

Directions:
1.   Preheat the breakfast sandwich maker.
2.   Place one of the tortillas inside the bottom tray of the sandwich maker. Brush with BBQ sauce.
3.   Break the pieces of bacon in half and place them on top of the tortilla. Sprinkle with cheese, red onion and red pepper.
4.   Slide the egg tray into place and crack the egg into it. Use a fork to stir the egg, just breaking the yolk.
5.   Place the second tortilla on top of the egg.
6.   Close the sandwich maker and cook for 4 to 5 minutes until the egg is cooked through.
7.   Carefully rotate the egg tray out of the sandwich maker then open the sandwich maker.
8.   Remove the top tortilla and spread with salsa and sour cream. Replace the tortilla and enjoy your sandwich.

104.   Southwest Quesadilla

Servings: 1
Cooking Time: 4 Minutes
Ingredients:
- 2 small corn tortillas
- 3 slices avocado
- Sea salt and pepper
- 1 slice tomato
- 1 slice Monterey Jack cheese
- Fresh chopped cilantro
- 1 egg

Directions:
1.   Place one corn tortilla in the bottom of sandwich maker. Place avocado on top and sprinkle with sea salt and pepper. Then add tomato, cheese and sprinkle with cilantro.
2.   Lower the cooking plate and top ring; crack an egg into the egg plate and pierce to break the yolk. Place other corn tortilla on top and close the lid.
3.   Cook for 3 to 4 minutes or until egg is cooked through. Gently slide the egg plate out and remove quesadilla with a rubber spatula. Slice in half and serve.

105.   Berry Pancake

Servings: 1
Cooking Time: 3 – 4 Minutes
Ingredients:
- 1 Frozen Pancake
- ¼ cup chopped frozen Berries
- 1 tsp Sugar
- 1 tbsp Whipped Cream

Directions:
1.   Preheat the sandwich maker and grease it with some cooking spray.
2.   Place the pancake on top of the bottom ring.
3.   Arrange the berries over and sprinkle with the sugar.
4.   Close the lid and cook for 3 – 4 minutes.
5.   Open carefully and transfer to a plate.
6.   Top with the whipped cream and enjoy!
Nutrition Info: Calories 117 Total Fats 2g Carbs 23g Protein 2.3g Fiber 2g

106.   Dijon And Berry Chicken Panini

Servings: 4
Cooking Time: 6 Minutes
Ingredients:
- 4 Bakery Ciabatta rolls or French hamburger buns
- 2 tablespoons herb garlic butter, melted
- 1/3 cup fresh blackberries (about 6 berries)
- 1 tablespoon honey
- 1/2 cup stone-ground mustard
- 3.5 oz. Deli aged white cheddar cheese, shredded
- 1 medium red onion, coarsely chopped
- 1 cup fresh baby arugula, coarsely chopped
- 1 Deli rotisserie chicken, shredded

Directions:
1.   Slice the rolls in half horizontally. Mash the berries in a bowl, and mix with the honey and then mix in the mustard. In a separate bowl mix together the chicken, arugula, cheese, and onions.
2.   Spread butter on the outside of the bread. Spread the berry mixture on the inside of the bread. Put chicken mixture on the inside of the bottom piece of bread, and place the top piece of bread on the chicken.
3.   Cook the sandwiches for 6 minutes on medium heat, and make sure to flip halfway through. The bread should be brown, and the cheese should be melted.

107.   Pesto Cheese Sandwich

Servings: 2
Cooking Time: 10minutes
Ingredients:
- 4 Italian or French bread slices
- 3 tbsp. Pesto
- 2 red peppers, roasted
- 6 basil leaves, fresh
- 4 mozzarella slices, fresh
- 1 tbsp. Tomatoes, sun-dried
- 3 tbsp. Butter softened

Directions:
1.   Preheat the sandwich maker/Panini on medium-low.
2.   Make the sandwich by layering the ingredients on one slice of bread and place the second on top.
3.   Spread butter on both outer layers and cook on the Panini for 3 minutesutes.
4.   Let it rest for 1 minutes.
5.   Cut and serve.

108. Lamb And Havarti Grilled Cheese Panini

Servings: 1
Cooking Time: 8 Minutes
Ingredients:
- 2 slices thick hearty bread
- 1 tablespoon butter, room temperature
- 1/2 cup Havarti, shredded
- 1/4 cup leftover lamb, reheated
- sliced red onion
- handful of spinach
- 2 tablespoons tzatziki, room temperature

Directions:
1. Spread butter on one side of each piece of bread.
2. Place a layer of cheese down, then the lamb, spinach onions, and tzatziki on one piece of bread. Make sure it's not on the buttered side. Then top with the other piece of bread, making sure the buttered side is up.
3. Cook the sandwiches 8 minutes on medium heat, and make sure to flip halfway through. The bread should be brown, and the cheese should be melted.

109. Ham-mango Croissant

Servings: 1
Cooking Time: 5 Minutes
Ingredients:
- 1 small croissant, sliced in half
- 1 slice ham
- A few slices mango
- Dash of cayenne pepper
- 1 slice white cheddar cheese
- 1 egg
- Sea salt and pepper

Directions:
1. Place one croissant half into the bottom ring of breakfast sandwich maker, cut side up. Place ham and mango on top, and lightly sprinkle with cayenne pepper. Next place the cheddar cheese.
2. Lower the cooking plate and top ring; crack an egg into the egg plate and pierce to break the yolk. Season with sea salt and pepper. Top with other croissant half.
3. Close the cover and cook for 4 to 5 minutes or until egg is cooked and sandwich is warmed through. Carefully remove sandwich with a rubber spatula.

110. Vegetarian Boca Sandwich

Servings: 1
Cooking Time: 5 Minutes
Ingredients:
- 1 whole wheat thin sandwich bun, sliced
- 2 tsp. Dijon mustard
- 1 Boca burger patty
- 1 slice Swiss cheese
- 1 large egg, beaten
- 1 slice red onion
- 1 slice tomato

Directions:
1. Preheat the breakfast sandwich maker.
2. Place half of the sandwich bun, cut-side up, inside the bottom tray of the sandwich maker.
3. Brush the sandwich bun with Dijon mustard.
4. Top the sandwich bun with the Boca burger patty and Swiss cheese.
5. Slide the egg tray into place and pour the beaten egg into it.
6. Place the second half of the sandwich bun on top of the egg.
7. Close the sandwich maker and cook for 4 to 5 minutes until the egg is cooked through.
8. Carefully rotate the egg tray out of the sandwich maker then open the sandwich maker.
9. Remove the top of the sandwich bun and top the sandwich with the red onion and tomato.
10. Replace the sandwich bun top and enjoy your sandwich.

111. Cheddar And Bacon Omelet

Servings: 1
Cooking Time: 3-4 Minutes
Ingredients:
- 2 Large Eggs
- 2 tbsp cooked and crumbled Bacon
- 2 tbsp shredded Cheddar Cheese
- Salt and Pepper, to taste

Directions:
1. Preheat your Breakfast Sandwich Maker and grease it with some cooking spray.
2. Beat the eggs lightly.
3. When the green lights turn on, open the unit, and add half of the whisked eggs into the bottom ring.
4. Top with the cheese and bacon.
5. Add the rest of the eggs to the cooking plate.
6. Close and cook for 3 to 4 minutes.
7. Rotate the handle clockwise to open.
8. Remove with a plastic or silicone spatula.
9. Serve and enjoy!
Nutrition Info: Calories 348 Total Fats 26g Carbs 1.2 g Protein 24.5g Fiber 0g

112.   Corn Bowl With Tomato, Bacon, And Cheese

Servings: 1
Cooking Time: 3 ½ Minutes
Ingredients:
- 1 Corn Tortilla
- 1 tbsp chopped Tomatoes
- 2 Basil Slices, chopped
- 1 ounce shredded Cheddar Cheese
- 2 Bacon Slices, chopped

Directions:
1. Preheat the sandwich maker and grease it with some cooking spray.
2. Add the corn tortilla to the bottom ring, and press it well inside to make it look like a bowl.
3. Add the rest of the ingredients inside.
4. Close the unit and cook for 3 ½ minutes.
5. Lift up to open and carefully transfer to a plate.
6. Serve and enjoy!

Nutrition Info: Calories 262 Total Fats 16.4g Carbs 13g Protein 16g Fiber 1.9g

113.   Easy Ham And Scrambled Egg

Servings: 1
Cooking Time: 5 Minutes
Ingredients:
- 2 slices whole grain bread
- 2 slices deli ham
- 1 slice Swiss cheese
- 1 large egg
- 2 teaspoons heavy cream
- 1 teaspoon chopped chives

Directions:
1. Preheat the breakfast sandwich maker.
2. Place one slice of bread in the bottom tray of the sandwich maker.
3. Arrange the slices of ham on top of the bread and top with the slice of Swiss cheese.
4. Beat together the egg, heavy cream and chives in a small bowl.
5. Slide the egg tray into place over the cheese and pour the beaten egg mixture into the tray.
6. Top the egg mixture with the remaining slice of bread.
7. Close the sandwich maker and cook for 4 to 5 minutes until the egg is cooked through.
8. Carefully rotate the egg tray out of the sandwich maker then open the sandwich maker and enjoy your sandwich.

114.   Tomato-basil With Mozzarella Sandwich

Servings: 1
Cooking Time: 5 Minutes
Ingredients:
- 2 slices specialty bread such as focaccia or sour dough
- 2 slices tomato
- A few fresh basil leaves
- 1 – 2 slices fresh mozzarella
- A few drops of balsamic vinegar
- 1 egg
- Sea salt and pepper

Directions:
1.   Place one slice of bread into the bottom ring of breakfast sandwich maker. Place tomatoes, basil and mozzarella cheese on top. Sprinkle with balsamic vinegar.
2.   Lower the cooking plate and top ring; crack an egg into the egg plate and pierce to break the yolk. Sprinkle with sea salt and pepper and top with other slice of bread.
3.   Close the cover and cook for 4 to 5 minutes or until egg is cooked through. Gently slide the egg plate out and remove sandwich with a rubber spatula. Slice in half and enjoy!

115.   Shaved Asparagus And Balsamic Cherries With Pistachios Panini

Servings: 4
Cooking Time: 6 Minutes
Ingredients:
- 1 to 1 and 1/2 cups pitted, chopped Bing cherries
- zest from 2 lemons
- 3 to 4 tbsp. balsamic vinegar
- roughly 1/2 bunch of thick-stalk asparagus, shaved with a mandolin or vegetable peeler
- 2 tbsp. fresh mint, thinly sliced
- 2 tbsp. fresh basil, thinly sliced
- 2 tbsp. pistachio oil
- 1 multigrain baguette, cut in half, and split open
- ricotta
- fresh mozzarella
- salt and freshly-cracked pepper
- 1/2 tbsp. butter, softened

Directions:
1.   Mix the cherries, balsamic vinegar, and lemon zest. Then salt and pepper to taste.
2.   Mix the asparagus mint, pistachio oil, and basil in a different bowl.
3.   Cut the mozzarella into slices that are 1/3 of an inch thick. Place them on the inside part of the pieces of bread and place the cherry mixture on top of it. Then place the asparagus mixture on top of that
4.   Use a knife top spread the ricotta on the inside of the top pieces of bread, and place it on the asparagus mixture.
5.   Cook the Panini on medium heat for 5 to 6 minutes, flipping halfway through. The bread should be brown, and the cheese should be melted.
6.   Cut the sandwiches in half before serving.

116.   Cuban Sandwich

Servings: 2
Cooking Time: 10minutes
Ingredients:
- 2 soft sandwich rolls, slice them lengthwise
- Mustard
- 1 dill pickle, sliced lengthwise
- 4 oz. sliced roast turkey
- 4 oz. sliced ham
- 3 oz. Provolone or Swiss cheese
- Softened Butter

Directions:
1. Spread the rolls with mustard. Now layer ½ of the ingredients, cheese, ham, turkey and pickle on each roll. Press them together. Spread the outside with butter.
2. Grill using the Panini for 5 minutes.
3. Serve and enjoy!

117.   Sausage And Cheese

Servings: 1
Cooking Time: 5 Minutes
Ingredients:
- 1 buttermilk biscuit, sliced
- 1 maple pork sausage patty, cooked
- 1 slice cheddar cheese
- 1 large egg, beaten

Directions:
1. Preheat the breakfast sandwich maker.
2. Place half of the biscuit, cut-side up, inside the bottom tray of the sandwich maker.
3. Arrange the sausage patty on top of the biscuit and top with the slice of cheddar cheese.
4. Slide the egg tray into place and pour the beaten egg into it.
5. Top the egg with the other half of the biscuit.
6. Close the sandwich maker and cook for 4 to 5 minutes until the egg is cooked through.
7. Carefully rotate the egg tray out of the sandwich maker then open the sandwich maker and enjoy your sandwich.

118.   Crunchy Nutella And Strawberry Bagel

Servings: 1
Cooking Time: 3 Minutes
Ingredients:
- ½ Bagel
- 1 tbsp Nutella
- 4 Strawberries, sliced
- 1 tsp chopped Hazelnuts

Directions:
1. Preheat the Hamilton Beach Breakfast Sandwich Maker until the green light appears. Spray with some cooking spray.
2. Spread the Nutella over the bagel.
3. Place the bagel on top of the bottom ring, with the cut-side up.
4. Arrange the strawberry slices over, and sprinkle with the hazelnuts.
5. Close the lid and cook for 3 minutes.
6. Rotate the handle clockwise to open.
7. Serve and enjoy!
Nutrition Info: Calories 220 Total Fats 8g Carbs 32g Protein 5.8g Fiber 2.2g

119.   Traditional Blt

Servings: 1
Cooking Time: 5 Minutes
Ingredients:
- 2 slices white bread
- 3 slices bacon, cooked
- 2 thin slices tomato
- 1 leaf Romaine lettuce, torn in half
- 2 teaspoons mayonnaise

Directions:
1. Spread one teaspoon of mayonnaise on each slice of bread.
2. Preheat the breakfast sandwich maker.
3. Place one slice of bread inside the bottom tray of the sandwich maker, mayonnaise-side facing up.
4. Break the slices of bacon in half and place them on top of the bread. Top with the slices of tomato.
5. Top the sandwich with the other slice of bread, mayonnaise-side down.
6. Close the sandwich maker and cook for 4 to 5 minutes.
7. Carefully open the sandwich maker and remove the top slice of bread.
8. Add the lettuce then replace the bread and enjoy your sandwich.

120.   Gluten-free Smoked Salmon And Cream Cheese Sandwich

Servings: 1
Cooking Time: 3 Minutes
Ingredients:
- 1 ounce Smoked Salmon
- 1 tbsp Cream Cheese
- 1 ounce shredded Mozzarella
- 2 gluten-free Bread Slices

Directions:
1. Preheat the sandwich maker and grease it with some cooking spray.
2. Cut the bread slices into circles that can fit inside the appliance.
3. When the green light appears, add one bread slice to the bottom ring.
4. Add half of the cream cheese and lightly spread it.
5. Add the smoked salmon and mozzarella on top.
6. Lower the top ring.
7. Spread the remaining cream cheese over the second bread slice.
8. Place the bread slice on top, with the cream cheese down.
9. Close the unit and cook for 3 minutes.
10. Rotate clockwise to open.
11. Serve and enjoy!

Nutrition Info: Calories 348 Total Fats 14.6g Carbs 39g Protein 15g Fiber 5g

121.   Eggs Benedict With Ham

Servings: 1
Cooking Time: 5 Minutes
Ingredients:
- 4 tablespoons unsalted butter
- 1 large egg yolk
- 2 teaspoons lemon juice
- Pinch cayenne pepper
- Pinch salt
- 1 whole wheat bagel, sliced
- ½ cup fresh spinach leaves
- 2 slices cooked bacon
- 1 large egg, beaten

Directions:
1. Preheat the breakfast sandwich maker.
2. Melt the butter in a small saucepan over medium heat.
3. Blend the egg yolks, lemon juice, cayenne and salt in a blender then drizzle into the saucepan.
4. Cook for 10 seconds, stirring well, then remove from heat and set aside.
5. Place half of the bagel, cut-side up, inside the bottom tray of the sandwich maker.
6. Top the bagel half with spinach leaves. Break the bacon slices in half and place them on top of the spinach.
7. Slide the egg tray into place and pour the beaten egg into it.
8. Top the egg with the other half of the bagel.
9. Close the sandwich maker and cook for 4 to 5 minutes until the egg is cooked through.
10. Carefully rotate the egg tray out of the sandwich maker then open the sandwich maker.
11. Take the top bagel off the sandwich and drizzle the eggs with the hollandaise sauce.
12. Replace the bagel half and enjoy your sandwich.

122.   Tropical Croissant With Sugar

Servings: 1
Cooking Time: 4 Minutes
Ingredients:
- 1 tbsp mashed canned Pineapple
- 1 tbsp Mango chunks
- 1 tsp Butter
- ½ Croissant
- 1 tsp Powdered Sugar

Directions:
1. Preheat the unit and grease it with cooking spray.
2. Spread the butter over the croissant, and place on top of the bottom ring, with the butter-side down.
3. Top with the pineapple and mango chunks.
4. Close the lid and cook for 3 minutes.
5. Rotate clockwise, and lift to open carefully.
6. Transfer to a plate and sprinkle with the powdered sugar.
7. Enjoy!

Nutrition Info: Calories 194 Total Fats 10g Carbs 24.6g Protein 2.6g Fiber 1.3g

123.   Eggs Benedict Sandwich

Servings: 1
Cooking Time: 4 To 5 Minutes
Ingredients:
- 4 Baby Spinach Leaves
- 1 English Muffin
- 1 Slice Canadian Bacon
- 1 tbsp Hollandaise Sauce
- 1 Egg, lightly whisked

Directions:
1. Preheat the Hamilton Beach Breakfast Sandwich Maker and spray it with some cooking spray.
2. Split the muffin in half and add one half to the bottom ring.
3. Top with the baby spinach and bacon.
4. Lower the cooking plate and add the egg to it.
5. Top with the remaining muffin half and close the unit.
6. Let cook for 4 to 5 minutes.
7. Turn the handle clockwise and open carefully.
8. Transfer the sandwich with a plastic spatula to a plate.
9. Drizzle the Hollandaise Sauce on top.
10. Enjoy!

Nutrition Info: Calories 330 Total Fats 14.7g Carbs 31g Protein 19g Fiber 2.5g

124.   Moist Leftover Chicken Biscuit

Servings: 1
Cooking Time: 4 Minutes
Ingredients:
- 1 Biscuit
- 2 ounces Leftover Chicken
- 2 tsp Heavy Cream
- 1 ounce shredded Cheddar Cheese

Directions:
1. Preheat the unit and grease it with cooking spray.
2. Cut the biscuit in half and add one half to the bottom ring, cut-side up.
3. Add the chicken and sprinkle the heavy cream over.
4. Top with the cheddar cheese and lower the top ring.
5. Add the second half of the biscuit, this time with the cut-side down, and close the unit.
6. Cook for 4 minutes.
7. Lift the lid and transfer the sandwich to a plate.
8. Serve and enjoy!

Nutrition Info: Calories 280 Total Fats 16g Carbs 12g Protein 22g Fiber 0.4g

125. Fried Egg And Cheese Bagel

Servings: 1
Cooking Time: 5 Minutes
Ingredients:
- 1 poppy seed bagel, sliced
- 1 ounce goat cheese
- 1 large egg
- 1 teaspoon chopped chives
- Salt and pepper to taste

Directions:
1. Preheat the breakfast sandwich maker.
2. Place half of the bagel, cut-side up, inside the bottom tray of the sandwich maker.
3. Layer the goat cheese on top of the bagel.
4. Slide the egg tray into place and crack the egg into it.
5. Sprinkle the egg with chopped chives, salt and pepper.
6. Top the egg with the other half of the bagel.
7. Close the sandwich maker and cook for 4 to 5 minutes until the egg is cooked through.
8. Carefully rotate the egg tray out of the sandwich maker then open the sandwich maker and enjoy your sandwich.

126. Creamy Strawberry Mint Croissant

Servings: 1
Cooking Time: 3 Minutes
Ingredients:
- 1 small croissant, sliced in half
- 1 Tbsp. cream cheese
- 1 Tbsp. strawberry jam
- 1 – 2 fresh strawberries, sliced
- A few fresh mint leaves

Directions:
1. Spread cream cheese and strawberry jam on both halves of croissant. Place one half in the bottom of breakfast sandwich maker, jam side up. Place strawberry slices on top, followed by a few fresh mint leaves.
2. Lower the cooking plate and top ring. Place other half of croissant on top and close the sandwich maker lid. Cook for 2 – 3 minutes or until the croissant is warmed through. Carefully remove from sandwich maker.

127. Canadian Bacon Bagel Sandwich

Servings: 1
Cooking Time: 5 Minutes
Ingredients:
- 1 sesame seed bagel, cut in half
- 2 slices Canadian bacon
- 1 slice cheddar cheese
- 1 large egg

Directions:
1. Preheat the breakfast sandwich maker.
2. Place half of the bagel, cut-side up, inside the bottom tray of the sandwich maker.
3. Arrange the slices of Canadian bacon on top of the bagel and top with the slice of cheddar cheese.
4. Slide the egg tray into place and crack the egg into it.
5. Top the egg with the other half of the bagel.
6. Close the sandwich maker and cook for 4 to 5 minutes until the egg is cooked through.
7. Carefully rotate the egg tray out of the sandwich maker then open the sandwich maker and enjoy your sandwich.

128.   Buffalo Chicken Panini

Servings: 4
Cooking Time: 4 Minutes
Ingredients:
- 2 cups shredded cooked chicken
- 1 large sweet onion, sliced
- 8 slices seedless rye
- 1/4 pound thinly sliced Swiss cheese, about 8 slices
- 1/4 cup blue cheese dressing
- 1 cup mayonnaise
- 1 cup buffalo hot sauce
- 2 tablespoons unsalted butter
- blue cheese dressing

Directions:
1.   Melt the butter in a large skillet on medium heat. Add the onions and cook for about 20 minutes.
2.   Mix the buffalo sauce and mayonnaise in a medium bowl and toss with the chicken.
3.   Put a slice of cheese on a piece of bread then the chicken, the onions and top with another slice of cheese and top with another piece of bread. Repeat the process with the remaining sandwiches. Spread the butter on the top and bottom of the sandwich
4.   Cook the sandwiches for 4 minutes on medium heat, and make sure to flip halfway through. The bread should be brown, and the cheese should be melted. Serve the sandwiches with a side of the blue cheese dressing.

129.   Mexican Gluten-free Pork Sandwich

Servings: 1
Cooking Time: 4 Minutes
Ingredients:
- 2 Corn Tortillas
- 2 ounces pulled Pork
- 2 tsp Salsa
- ½ tbsp Beans
- 1 tsp Corn
- 1 Tomato Slice, chopped
- 2 tsp Red Onion
- 2 tbsp shredded Cheddar Cheese

Directions:
1.   Preheat the sandwich maker and grease it with some cooking spray.
2.   Cut the corn tortillas into 4-inch circles to fit inside the unit.
3.   Place one tortilla to the bottom ring and place the pork on top.
4.   Add the salsa, corn, beans, onion, and tomato, and top with the shredded cheese.
5.   Lower the top ring and add the second corn tortilla.
6.   Close and cook for 3-4 minutes.
7.   Rotate clockwise and open carefully.
8.   Transfer to a plate.
9.   Serve and enjoy!
Nutrition Info: Calories 360 Total Fats 25g Carbs 21g Protein 24g Fiber 5g

130.   Pork Sandwiches

Servings: 10
Cooking Time: 6 Hours
Ingredients:
- 1 Onion, sliced
- ¾ cup Chicken broth, reduced-sodium
- 1 cup Parsley, minutesced
- 7 cloves of garlic, minutesced
- 2 tbsp. Cider Vinegar
- 1 tbsp. lemon juice + 1 ½ tsp.
- 2 tsp. Cuminutes, ground
- 1 tsp. Mustard, ground
- 1 tsp. oregano, dried
- ½ tsp. of Salt
- ½ tsp. Black pepper
- 1 (4 lb.) Pork shoulder, boneless
- 1 ¼ cups Mayo, fat-free
- 2 tbsp. Dijon mustard
- 10 Hamburger buns
- 1 ¼ cups of shredded Swiss cheese
- 1 Onion, sliced into rings
- 2 dill pickles, whole, sliced

Directions:
1.   Prepare the pork the night before. Place the broth and onion in a slow cooker. In a bowl combine black pepper, salt, oregano, mustard, cuminutes, lemon juice, vinegar, 5 cloves of garlic and parsley. Stir well and rub the pork. Add in the cooker and cook 6-8 hours.
2.   Remove the meat and let it rest for about 10 minutes before you slice it.
3.   In a bowl combine the remaining lemon and garlic, mustard and mayo. Spread over the buns (split the buns). Layer the bottom buns with pickles, onions, cheese, and pork. Top with half-bun.
4.   Cook on a sandwich maker for about 3 minutes.
5.   Serve and enjoy!

131.   Spicy Turkey And Sausage Sandwich

Servings: 1
Cooking Time: 4 Minutes
Ingredients:
- 1 ounce cooked ground Turkey
- 4 slices of Spicy Sausage
- 2 tsp Salsa
- ¼ tsp Cumin
- 1 tbsp refined Beans
- 1 tsp Sour Cream
- 1 tbsp shredded Cheddar Cheese
- 2 small Tortillas

Directions:
1.   Preheat the sandwich maker and grease it with some cooking spray.
2.   Cut the tortillas into circles so they can fit inside the unit.
3.   Add one tortilla on top of the bottom ring and spread half of the salsa over.
4.   Top with the turkey and sausage, and sprinkle the cumin over.
5.   Add the beans and cheese, and drizzle the sour cream over.
6.   Brush the remaining salsa on the second tortilla and place it on top of the cheese with the salsa-side down.
7.   Close the unit and cook for 4 minutes.
8.   Lift it open and transfer to a plate carefully.
9.   Serve and enjoy!
Nutrition Info: Calories 470 Total Fats 26g Carbs 32g Protein 26g Fiber 3g

132.   Herbed Omelet With Cream Cheese And Cheddar

Servings: 1
Cooking Time: 4-5 Minutes
Ingredients:
- 1 ounce Shredded Cheddar
- 2 Eggs
- ¼ tsp Garlic Powder
- 2 tsp Cream Cheese
- 1 tsp chopped Parsley
- 1 tsp chopped Cilantro
- ½ tsp chopped Dill
- Pinch of Smoked Paprika
- Salt and Pepper, to taste

Directions:
1. Preheat and grease the sandwich maker.
2. Whisk the eggs and season with salt, pepper, garlic powder, and paprika.
3. Stir in the cream cheese, parsley, and cilantro.
4. When the green light appears, pour half of the eggs into the bottom ring of the unit.
5. Top with the shredded cheddar and dill.
6. Lower the top ring and cooking plate, and pour the remaining eggs inside.
7. Close the unit and let cook for 4 to 5 minutes.
8. Rotate the handle clockwise and transfer to a plate.
9. Serve as desired and enjoy!

Nutrition Info: Calories 290 Total Fats 22g Carbs 1.8g Protein 20.5g Fiber 0.1g

133.   French Toast And Grilled Banana Panini

Servings: 4
Cooking Time: 6 Minutes
Ingredients:
- 6 large eggs
- 1 cup whole milk
- 1/2 cup heavy cream
- 1/4 cup fresh orange juice (from about 1 medium orange)
- 2 tablespoons vanilla extract
- 2 tablespoons cognac (optional)
- 2 tablespoons granulated sugar
- 1/2 teaspoon ground cinnamon
- Pinch of freshly grated nutmeg
- Salt
- 8 slices Texas toast or other thick white bread
- 3 large ripe bananas
- 2 tablespoons unsalted butter, melted
- Confectioners' sugar, for garnish
- Pure maple syrup, for garnish

Directions:
1. Use a whisk to combine the eggs, milk, cream, orange juice, cognac, sugar, cinnamon, and vanilla. Put the bread in a couple of shallow baking dishes and cover with the mixture you just created. Allow the bread to rest in the mixture for 10 minutes
2. While the bread is resting preheat a skillet on medium heat. Then coat the bananas with melted butter and cook them in the skillet until are nice and brown all over, about 3 minutes. They should be releasing their juices. When bananas have cooled down a little chop them into chunks.
3. Preheat your flip sandwich maker on medium high heat. While that's preheating place the bananas on half the pieces of bread and top with the other pieces of bread.
4. Cook the Panini for 6 to 7 minutes in your preheated flap sandwiched maker, flipping halfway through.
5. Top with confectioners' sugar and maple syrup

134.   Prosciutto And Egg Bagel Panini

Servings: 2
Cooking Time: 3 Minutes
Ingredients:

- 2 eggs
- 2 everything bagels (or any favorite bagel)
- 2 tablespoons mayonnaise
- 2 slices American cheese
- 4 slices prosciutto
- 2 handfuls baby arugula
- Kosher salt
- Ground black pepper
- Olive oil
- 2 teaspoon butter

Directions:

1. Use a whisk to beat the egg with a pinch of salt and pepper. Place the butter in a skillet and melt it on medium heat. Use a spoon to stir the eggs and push them across the pan. Cook until the eggs set, about 1 to 20 minutes.
2. Cut the bagels in half horizontally. Spread the mayonnaise on the inside of the bagel. Layer the eggs, on the inside of 2 of the bagel halves, then the cheese, then the arugula, then the prosciutto. Top with the remaining pieces of bagel. Brush the top and bottom of the sandwiches with olive oil.
3. Cook the Panini on medium heat for 2 to 3 minutes, flipping halfway through. The bagels should be toasted, and the cheese should be melted.

135.   Apple Pie Sandwich

Servings: 4
Cooking Time: 5 Minutes
Ingredients:

- ½ cup of Mascarpone Cheese
- 2 tsp. Honey
- 4 tbsp. room temperature butter
- 8 slices of Cinnamon bread
- 1 apple, Granny Smith, cored and then sliced thinly
- 2 tbsp. Brown sugar, light

Directions:

1. In a bowl combine the honey and mascarpone. Whisk until fluffy and smooth.
2. Turn on medium-high heat and preheat the sandwich maker.
3. Spread butter on 2 bread slices. Flip them and spread 1 tbsp. of the mascarpone. Top with apple slices and close with the other bread slices.
4. Sprinkle with brown sugar.
5. Grill for 5 minutes.
6. Serve and enjoy!

136.   The Thanksgiving Turkey Cuban Panini

Servings: 4
Cooking Time: 7 Minutes
Ingredients:
- 2 tablespoons mayonnaise
- 2 tablespoons Dijon mustard
- 2 tablespoons leftover cranberry sauce
- Salt and freshly ground black pepper
- 4 slices good quality Italian bread
- 4 slices Swiss cheese
- 2 slices cooked ham
- 6 slices leftover cooked turkey
- 8 dill pickle slices
- Olive oil

Directions:
1.   Mix together the first mayonnaise, cranberry sauce, and Dijon mustard using a whisk. Salt and pepper to taste. Combine the mixture with the cabbage until well coated.
2.   Spread a layer of the newly made cranberry Dijon sauce on what's going to be the inside of 2 pieces of bread. Put a layer of cheese, then turkey, a layer of the ham, a layer of pickles, and another layer of cheese on the pieces of bread. Top with another piece of bread. Brush the top and bottom of the sandwich with olive oil
3.   Cook the sandwiches for 6 to 7 minutes on medium high heat, and make sure to flip halfway through. The bread should be toasted, and the cheese should be melted. Once you're ready to serve, slice the sandwiches in half.

137.   Breakfast Pizza Sandwich

Servings: 1
Cooking Time: 5 Minutes
Ingredients:
- 2 pieces pita bread, cut to fit sandwich maker
- 2 Tbsp. store bought marinara sauce
- 1 slice ham
- A few slices of pepperoni
- Basil leaves
- 1 – 2 slices mozzarella cheese
- 1 egg

Directions:
1.   Spread marinara sauce on both pieces of pita bread. Place one piece into the bottom ring of breakfast sandwich maker, marinara side up. Place ham, pepperoni, basil and mozzarella cheese on top.
2.   Lower the cooking plate and top ring; crack an egg into the egg plate and pierce to break the yolk. Top with other piece of pita bread.
3.   Close the cover and cook for 4 to 5 minutes or until egg is cooked through. Gently slide the egg plate out, remove sandwich with a rubber spatula and enjoy!

138.   Almond Butter & Honey Biscuit

Servings: 1
Cooking Time: 3 Minutes
Ingredients:
- 1 store bought or homemade biscuit, split
- 1 Tbsp. almond butter
- 1 – 2 tsp. honey
- Dash of cinnamon

Directions:
1.   Spread the almond butter on half of the biscuit and then drizzle honey on top. Place biscuit, almond butter side up, into the bottom ring of breakfast sandwich maker. Sprinkle with cinnamon.
2.   Lower the cooking plate and top ring and top with other biscuit half. Close the cover and cook for 3 to 4 minutes or until biscuit is warmed through. Remove sandwich with a rubber spatula.

139.   Lamb Panini Burger

Servings: 8
Cooking Time: 10 Minutes
Ingredients:
- 2 1/2 pounds ground lamb, preferably shoulder
- 1 medium onion, very finely chopped
- 3/4 cup chopped fresh flat-leaf parsley
- 1 tablespoon ground coriander
- 3/4 teaspoon ground cumin
- 1/2 teaspoon ground cinnamon
- 2 teaspoons kosher salt
- 1 1/2 teaspoons freshly ground black pepper
- 1/4 cup olive oil, plus more for grilling
- 8 thick medium pita breads with pockets

Directions:
1.   Combine the lamb, oil, and seasoning using a fork. Allow the meat to rest, covered for an hour.
2.   Open up the pitas and fill them with the lamb mixture. Use the fill the seal the pita.
3.   Cook the sandwiches for 10 minutes on medium heat, and make sure to flip halfway through. The bread should be nicely crunchy and the lamb is cooked through.

140.   Chili Cheesy Omelet With Bacon

Servings: 1
Cooking Time: 4 ½ Minutes
Ingredients:
- 2 Eggs, whisked
- 1/4 Red Chili, chopped
- ¼ tsp Garlic Powder
- 1 slice cooked and crumbled Bacon
- 1 ounce Mozzarella Cheese, shredded
- Salt and Pepper, to taste

Directions:
1.   Preheat and grease the sandwich maker.
2.   Season the eggs with salt, pepper, and garlic powder.
3.   When the green light appears, add half of the whisked eggs to the bottom ring.
4.   Place the mozzarella, bacon, and chilli on top.
5.   Add the remaining eggs to the cooking plate.
6.   Close and let cook for 4 ½ minutes.
7.   Open by sliding clockwise and transfer the omelet carefully to a plate.
8.   Serve and enjoy!

Nutrition Info: Calories 277 Total Fats 18g Carbs 2.8g Protein 24.7g Fiber 2.8g

141. Blueberry Waffle Sandwich

Servings: 1
Cooking Time: 5 Minutes
Ingredients:
- 2 small store bought frozen blueberry waffles
- Butter
- 2 strips bacon
- 1 slice cheddar cheese
- 1 egg
- Sea salt and pepper

Directions:
1. Spread butter on both waffles. Place one into the bottom ring of breakfast sandwich maker, butter side down. Place bacon and cheddar cheese on top.
2. Lower the cooking plate and top ring; crack an egg into the egg plate and pierce to break the yolk. Season with sea salt and pepper. Top with other waffle.
3. Close the cover and cook for 4 to 5 minutes or until egg is cooked and cheese is melted. Remove sandwich with a rubber spatula.

142. Cornbread And Egg Sandwich

Servings: 1
Cooking Time: 4 Minutes
Ingredients:
- 2 corn-only Cornbread Slices
- 1 Egg
- 1 tbsp shredded Cheddar
- 1 tsp cooked and crumbled Bacon

Directions:
1. Preheat the unit and grease it with some cooking spray.
2. Cut the cornbread slcies into rounds so they can fit inside the unit, and place one on top of the bottom ring.
3. Add the cheddar and bacon.
4. Whisk the egg a bit, lower the cooking plate, and add it to it.
5. Place the second cornbread slice on top.
6. Close the sandwich maker and cook for 4 minutes.
7. Slide out and open the lid carefully.
8. Transfer to a plate and enjoy!

Nutrition Info: Calories 320 Total Fats 17g Carbs 24g Protein 12g Fiber 4g

143.   Mediterranean Croissant

Servings: 1
Cooking Time: 5 Minutes
Ingredients:
- 1 small croissant, sliced in half
- 1 Tbsp. store bought pesto
- 1 Tbsp. sun-dried tomatoes
- Baby spinach leaves
- 1 slice havarti cheese
- 1 egg

Directions:
1.   Spread pesto on both croissant halves. Place one half into the bottom ring of breakfast sandwich maker, pesto side up. Place sun-dried tomatoes, a few spinach leaves and havarti cheese on top.
2.   Lower the cooking plate and top ring; crack an egg into the egg plate and pierce to break the yolk. Top with other croissant half.
3.   Close the cover and cook for 4 to 5 minutes or until egg is cooked through and cheese is melted. Gently slide the egg plate out and remove sandwich with a rubber spatula.

144.   Canned Salmon And Bacon Pickle Sandwich

Servings: 1
Cooking Time: 3-4 Minutes
Ingredients:
- 2 ounces canned Salmon
- 1 Bacon Slice, cooked
- 2 Bread Slices
- 1 ounce shredded Mozzarella Cheese
- 1 tsp Pickle Relish
- ½ Pickle, sliced
- 1 tsp Dijon Mustard
- 1 tsp Tomato Puree

Directions:
1.   Preheat the sandwich maker and grease it with some cooking spray.
2.   Cut the bread slices so they can fit the unit.
3.   Brush one of the bread slices with Dijon mustard and place it on top oh the bottom ring, with the mustard-side up.
4.   Add the salmon and bacon on top and sprinkle with the relish and tomato puree.
5.   Arrange the pickle slices over and top with the mozzarella.
6.   Lower the top ring and add the second bread slice.
7.   Cover the unit and cook for about 3-4 minutes.
8.   Rotate clockwise to open an transfer to a plate.
9.   Serve and enjoy!
Nutrition Info: Calories 420 Total Fats 34g Carbs 25g Protein 28g Fiber 3.5g

145.   Tilapia And Pimento Dijon Sandwich

Servings: 1
Cooking Time: 3-4 Minutes
Ingredients:
- 2 Bread Slices
- 2 ounces chopped cooked Tilapia Fillet
- 1 slice Pimento Cheese
- 2 tsp Dijon Mustard
- ¼ tsp chopped Parsley

Directions:
1. Preheat the sandwich maker and grease it with some cooking spray.
2. Cut the bread slices so they can fit inside the unit, and brush the Dijon over them.
3. Place one bread slice into the bottom ring, with the mustard-side up.
4. Add the tilapia, sprinkle with parsley, and top with cheese.
5. Lower the ring and add the second bread slice, with the mustard-side down.
6. Close the appliance and cook for 3 to 4 minutes.
7. Open carefully and transfer to a plate.
8. Serve and enjoy!

Nutrition Info: Calories 388 Total Fats 13g Carbs 35g Protein 29g Fiber 6g

146.   Bahn Mi Panini

Servings: 1
Cooking Time: 4 Minutes
Ingredients:
- 1 petite baguette roll or 7-inch section from a regular baguette
- Mayonnaise
- Maggi Seasoning sauce or light (regular) soy sauce
- Liver pâté, boldly flavored cooked pork, sliced and at room temperature
- 3 or 4 thin, seeded cucumber strips, preferably English
- 2 or 3 sprigs cilantro, coarsely chopped
- 3 or 4 thin slices jalapeno chili
- 1/4 cup Daikon and Carrot Pickle

Directions:
1. Cut the bread in half lengthwise. Use your fingers to take out some of the soft part of the middle of both pieces of bread.
2. Spread the mayonnaise inside both pieces of bread. Lightly coat with the Maggi seasoning sauce, then place the meat on top followed by the cucumbers, cilantro, jalapenos, and then pickles.
3. Cook the Panini on medium heat for 4 minutes, flipping halfway through. The bread should be nicely toasted.

147.   Peach Coconut Cream Croissant

Servings: 1
Cooking Time: 3 Minutes
Ingredients:
- 1 small croissant, sliced in half
- 1 Tbsp. cream cheese
- 1 Tbsp. peach jam
- 3 – 4 fresh peach slices
- Shredded coconut
- Dash of cinnamon and nutmeg

Directions:
1.   Spread cream cheese and peach jam on both halves of croissant. Place one half in the bottom of breakfast sandwich maker, jam side up. Place peach slices on top. Sprinkle with some shredded coconut and a dash of cinnamon and nutmeg.
2.   Lower cooking plate and top ring. Place other half of croissant on top and close the sandwich maker lid. Cook for 2 – 3 minutes or until the croissant is warmed through. Carefully remove from sandwich maker and enjoy!

148.   Pork Muffin Sandwich

Servings: 1
Cooking Time: 5 Minutes
Ingredients:
- 1 Frozen Pork Pattie
- 1 English Muffin
- 1 Slice Cheddar Cheese
- 1 tsp Dijon Mustard

Directions:
1.   Preheat and grease the sandwich maker.
2.   Cut the muffin in half and brush one of the halves with the mustard.
3.   Place the muffin half onto the bottom ring with the mustard-side up.
4.   Top with the frozen pattie and place the cheese on top.
5.   Lower the top ring and add the second half with the cut-side down.
6.   Cook for full 5 minutes.
7.   Open by rotating clockwise and lifting the lid.
8.   Transfer to a plate and enjoy!

Nutrition Info: Calories 490 Total Fats 27g Carbs 25g Protein 33g Fiber 2g

Servings: 2
Cooking Time: 4 Minutes

Ingredients:

- 1 medium Avocado peeled and seeded
- ½ tablespoon Cilantro leaves finely chopped
- ½ teaspoon Lime juice
- Salt to taste
- Chipotle mayonnaise (store bought or homemade)
- 4 slices large Sourdough bread
- 8 slices Colby Jack Cheese
- 8 slices Blackened Oven Roasted Turkey Breast
- 4 slices Tomato

Directions:

1. Mash and mix the avocado, lime and cilantro, and then salt and pepper to taste.
2. Spread the chipotle mayonnaise on one side of every piece of bread. On 2 pieces of bread with the mayonnaise side facing up place a layer of cheese, then turkey, then tomato, then avocado mixture, then turkey, and finally cheese again. Top with another piece of bread with the mayonnaise side touching the cheese.
3. Cook the sandwiches for 6 minutes on medium heat, and make sure to flip halfway through. The bread should be toasted, and the cheese should be melted.

150.   The Ultimate Chicken, Spinach And Mozzarella Sandwich

Servings: 1
Cooking Time: 4 Minutes
Ingredients:
- 1 small Hamburger Bun
- 3 ounces cooked and chopped Chicken
- 1 tbsp Cream Cheese
- 1 ounce shredded Mozzarella
- 1 tbsp canned Corn
- 2 tbsp chopped Spinach

Directions:
1. Preheat and grease the sandwich maker.
2. Cut the bun in half and brush the cream cheese on the insides.
3. Add one half to the bottom ring, with the cut-side up.
4. Place the chicken on top and top with the spinach, corn, and mozzarella.
5. Lower the top ring and add the second half of the bun, the cut-side down.
6. Cook for 4 minutes.
7. Rotate clockwise and lift to open.
8. Serve and enjoy!

Nutrition Info: Calories 402 Total Fats 15.5g Carbs 32g Protein 32.5g Fiber 1.4g

151.   Mediterranean English Muffin

Servings: 1
Cooking Time: 5 Minutes
Ingredients:
- 1 English muffin, sliced
- 1 tsp. olive oil
- Salt and pepper to taste
- 1 ounce feta cheese crumbled
- 1 roasted red pepper in oil, drained
- 1 slice tomato
- 1 tbsp. basil pesto
- 1 large egg

Directions:
1. Preheat the breakfast sandwich maker.
2. Place half of the English muffin, cut-side up, inside the bottom tray of the sandwich maker.
3. Brush the English muffin with the olive oil and sprinkle with salt and pepper.
4. Top the muffin with the crumbled feta, roasted red pepper and tomato.
5. Slide the egg tray into place and crack the egg into it. Use a fork to stir the egg, just breaking the yolk.
6. Place the second half of the English muffin on top of the egg.
7. Close the sandwich maker and cook for 4 to 5 minutes until the egg is cooked through.
8. Carefully rotate the egg tray out of the sandwich maker then open the sandwich maker.
9. Remove the top English muffin and brush with basil pesto.
10. Replace the English muffin and enjoy your sandwich.

152.   Masala Sandwich

Servings: 1
Cooking Time: 5minutes
Ingredients:
- 2 slices of sandwich Bread
- 1 cucumber, sliced
- Margarine
- 1/3 red onion, small, sliced
- 1 Tomato, ripe, sliced
- Chaat Masala to taste

Directions:
1. First, spread margarine on the bread slices
2. Layer the veggies, start with the cucumber, tomatoes and then onion.
3. Sprinkle with chat masala.
4. Close the sandwich and grill on the Panini maker. Grill for 3 minutes.
5. Serve immediately and enjoy!

153.   Bacon Cheddar Croissant

Servings: 1
Cooking Time: 5 Minutes
Ingredients:
- 1 croissant, sliced
- 2 slices bacon, cooked
- 1 slice cheddar cheese
- 1 large egg, beaten

Directions:
1. Preheat the breakfast sandwich maker.
2. Place half of the croissant, cut-side up, inside the bottom tray of the sandwich maker.
3. Break the slices of bacon in half and arrange them on top of the croissant then top with the slice of cheddar cheese.
4. Slide the egg tray into place and pour the beaten egg into it.
5. Top the egg with the other half of the croissant.
6. Close the sandwich maker and cook for 4 to 5 minutes until the egg is cooked through.
7. Carefully rotate the egg tray out of the sandwich maker then open the sandwich maker and enjoy your sandwich.

154. Pancetta Cherry Tomato And Egg English Muffin Panini

Servings: 1
Cooking Time: 6 Minutes
Ingredients:
- 1 English muffin
- 1 egg
- 5 cherry tomatoes
- Fresh basil, chopped
- 2 slices of mozzarella
- Olive oil
- 1 teaspoon butter
- 4 thin slices of pancetta, cooked

Directions:
1. Use a whisk to beat the egg with a pinch of salt and pepper. Place the butter in a skillet and melt it on medium heat. Use a spoon to stir the eggs and push them across the pan. Cook until the eggs set, about 1 to 2 minutes.
2. Put a layer of avocado on the Harissa side of the 2 pieces of bread, then the sausage, then the arugula, and top with the cheese. Then place the other two pieces of bread on top of the cheese. Brush the top and bottom of the sandwiches with olive oil.
3. Cook the Panini on medium heat for 4 to 6 minutes, flipping halfway through. The bread should be toasted, and the cheese should be melted.

155. Sour Cream And Crab Cake Sandwich

Servings: 1
Cooking Time: 3 ½ Minutes
Ingredients:
- 1 frozen Crab Cake Pattie
- 2 tsp Sour Cream
- 1 slice American Cheese
- ½ Pickle, sliced
- 1 Biscuit

Directions:
1. Preheat the sandwich maker and grease it with some cooking spray.
2. Cut the biscuit in half and place one half to the bottom ring of the unit.
3. Spread half of the sour cream over and add the crab cake on top.
4. Spread the remaining sour cream over the crab cake, arrange the pickle slices over, and top with the cheese.
5. Lower the top ring and add the second biscuit half.
6. Close the unit and cook for 3 ½ minutes.
7. Open carefully and transfer to a plate.
8. Serve and enjoy!

Nutrition Info: Calories 340 Total Fats 26g Carbs 21g Protein 23g Fiber 3g

156.   Mixed Berry French Toast Panini

Servings: 4
Cooking Time: 6 Minutes
Ingredients:
- 6 large eggs
- 1 cup whole milk
- 1/2 cup heavy cream
- 1/4 cup fresh orange juice (from about 1 medium orange)
- 2 tablespoons vanilla extract
- 2 tablespoons cognac (optional)
- 2 tablespoons granulated sugar
- 1/2 teaspoon ground cinnamon
- Pinch of freshly grated nutmeg
- Salt
- 8 slices Texas toast or other thick white bread
- 1 cup blackberries
- 1 cup raspberries
- Confectioners' sugar, for garnish
- Pure maple syrup, for garnish

Directions:
1.   Spread the cream cheese on what's going to be the inside of the pieces of bread and then place the strawberries on top of 4 of them. Top with the remaining pieces of bread.
2.   Use a whisk to combine the eggs, milk, cream, orange juice, cognac, sugar, cinnamon, and vanilla. Put the sandwiches in a shallow baking dishes and cover with the mixture you just created. Allow sandwiches to rest in the mixture for 10 minutes.
3.   Preheat your flip sandwich maker on medium high heat.
4.   Cook the Panini for 6 to 7 minutes in your preheated flap sandwiched maker, flipping halfway through.
5.   Top with confectioners' sugar and maple syrup.

157.   Chocolate Raspberry Croissant

Servings: 1
Cooking Time: 5 Minutes
Ingredients:
- 1 croissant, sliced
- 2 tbsp. chocolate hazelnut spread
- ½ cup fresh raspberries
- 2 tbsp. crème fraiche

Directions:
1.   Brush 1 tbsp. chocolate hazelnut spread on each half of the croissant.
2.   Preheat the breakfast sandwich maker.
3.   Place half of the croissant, cut-side up, inside the bottom tray of the sandwich maker.
4.   Top the croissant with the raspberries and crème fraiche.
5.   Place the second half of the croissant on top of the raspberries.
6.   Close the sandwich maker and cook for 4 to 5 minutes until heated through.
7.   Carefully open the sandwich maker and enjoy your sandwich.

158.   Mushroom & Swiss Bagel

Servings: 1
Cooking Time: 10 Minutes
Ingredients:
- 1 multigrain bagel, split
- 2 large mushrooms, sliced
- 1 tsp. butter
- Sea salt and pepper
- 1 slice Swiss cheese
- 1 egg

Directions:
1. Place one bagel half, cut side up into the bottom ring of breakfast sandwich maker.
2. In a small skillet over medium heat, sauté mushrooms in butter until they shrink and begin to let out moisture. Season with sea salt and pepper. Place mushrooms on top of bagel and cover with Swiss cheese.
3. Lower the cooking plate and top ring; crack an egg into the egg plate and pierce to break the yolk. Top with other bagel half.
4. Close the cover and cook for 4 to 5 minutes or until egg is cooked through. Gently slide the egg plate out and remove sandwich with a rubber spatula.

159.   Corn And Zucchini Pepper Jack Panini

Servings: 4
Cooking Time: 10 Minutes
Ingredients:
- 1 tablespoon olive oil
- 1 large clove garlic, minced
- 1 ear corn, kernels removed
- 1 small zucchini, quartered lengthwise and sliced
- Salt + pepper to taste
- 8 slices bread
- 2 tbsp. butter, softened
- 1 cup shredded pepper jack cheese

Directions:
1. Place the oil in a skillet and heat it on medium high heat. Cook the garlic in the oil for about 15 seconds, until it's fragrant. Mix in the corn and zucchini and cook for around 3 minutes. The zucchini should be soft but not mushy. Remove the mixture from the heat and salt and pepper to taste.
2. Place a layer of cheese on 4 pieces of bread, then the vegetable mixture, and then another layer of cheese. Top with the remaining slices of bread. Butter both the top and bottom of the sandwich.
3. Cook the Panini on high heat for 5 to 7 minutes, flipping halfway through. The bread should be brown, and the cheese should be melted.

84

160.   Thai Breakfast Sandwich

Servings: 1
Cooking Time: 6 Minutes
Ingredients:
- 2 slices whole wheat bread
- 1 Tbsp. peanut butter
- 1 Tbsp. shredded carrots
- 1 Tbsp. bean sprouts
- 1 tsp. finely chopped cilantro
- Dash of lime juice
- Dash of soy sauce
- 1 Tbsp. milk
- 1 egg
- Sea salt and pepper

Directions:
1.   Spread peanut butter on both slices of bread. Place one slice into the bottom ring of breakfast sandwich maker, peanut butter side up. Pile the carrots, bean sprouts and cilantro on top. Sprinkle with lime juice and soy sauce.
2.   In a small bowl whisk together milk, egg, sea salt and pepper. Lower the cooking plate and top ring; pour egg mixture in. Top with other slice of bread.
3.   Close the cover and cook for 4 to 5 minutes or until egg is cooked. Remove sandwich with a rubber spatula.

161.   Ratatouille Panini

Servings: 1
Cooking Time: 16 Minutes
Ingredients:
- 1 red bell pepper, sliced
- 1 tomato, chopped
- 1 clove garlic, minced
- 1 teaspoon dried oregano, or to taste
- salt and ground black pepper to taste
- 1 eggplant, sliced
- 1 zucchini, sliced
- 1 tomato, sliced
- 1 red onion, sliced
- 4 teaspoons olive oil
- 4 slices sourdough bread
- 4 slices mozzarella cheese

Directions:
1.   Warm a skillet on high heat, and place the red bell pepper in it for around 5 minutes. The pepper should be soft when it's ready. Place the red pepper, chopped tomato, garlic in a blender or food processor. Blend or process until a smooth sauce is formed. Add salt, pepper, and oregano to taste.
2.   Grill the remaining vegetable on a grille or the same skillet for about 6 minutes flipping halfway through. The vegetables will be soft when ready.
3.   Brush what's going to be the outside of the bread slices with olive oil. Spread the sauce on what's going to be the inside of the bread. Layer a piece of piece of cheese on 2 of the pieces of bread, then the vegetable mixture, then another piece of cheese. Top with another piece of bread with the sauce side touching the cheese.
4.   Cook the Panini on medium heat for 4 to 5 minutes, flipping halfway through. The bread should be toasted, and the cheese should be melted.

162. Cinnamon Raisin Apple Sandwich

Servings: 1
Cooking Time: 5 Minutes
Ingredients:
- 2 slices cinnamon raisin bread
- ½ small apple, sliced thin
- 1 thin slice cheddar cheese
- ½ teaspoon unsalted butter
- Pinch ground cinnamon and nutmeg

Directions:
1. Preheat the breakfast sandwich maker.
2. Place one slice of bread inside the bottom tray of the sandwich maker. Spread the bread with butter.
3. Top the bread with the slices of apple then sprinkle them with cinnamon and nutmeg.
4. Place the slice of cheddar cheese over the apples. Top the cheese with the other piece of bread.
5. Close the sandwich maker and cook for 4 to 5 minutes until it is heated through.
6. Carefully open the sandwich maker and enjoy your sandwich.

163. Avocado Mash Sandwich

Servings: 1
Cooking Time: 8 Minutes
Ingredients:
- 2 slices French bread
- ½ small avocado
- 1 Tbsp. diced tomato
- ¼ tsp. garlic salt
- Black pepper
- 1 slice provolone cheese
- 1 egg

Directions:
1. Place one slice of French bread into the bottom ring of breakfast sandwich maker. In a small bowl, mash together avocado, tomato, garlic salt and pepper using a fork. Place avocado mixture on French bread slice and top with provolone cheese.
2. Lower the cooking plate and top ring; crack an egg into the egg plate and pierce to break the yolk. Top with other slice of French bread.
3. Close the cover and cook for 4 to 5 minutes or until egg is cooked through. Gently slide the egg plate out and remove sandwich with a rubber spatula.

164.   Blta (bacon, Lettuce, Tomato And Avocado)

Servings: 1
Cooking Time: 5 Minutes
Ingredients:
- 1 croissant, sliced in half
- 1 tablespoon mayonnaise
- Salt and pepper to taste
- 3 slices bacon, cooked
- ¼ ripe avocado, pitted and sliced
- 1 thick slice tomato
- 1 piece Romaine lettuce, torn in half
- 1 large egg

Directions:
1. Preheat the breakfast sandwich maker.
2. Place half of the croissant, cut-side up, inside the bottom tray of the sandwich maker.
3. Brush the croissant with the mayonnaise and sprinkle with salt and pepper.
4. Break the bacon slices in half and arrange them on top of the croissant. Top with avocado and tomato.
5. Slide the egg tray into place and crack the egg into it. Use a fork to stir the egg, just breaking the yolk.
6. Place the second half of the croissant on top of the egg.
7. Close the sandwich maker and cook for 4 to 5 minutes until the egg is cooked through.
8. Carefully rotate the egg tray out of the sandwich maker then open the sandwich maker.
9. Remove the top of the croissant and top with the lettuce.
10. Replace the top half of the croissant then enjoy your sandwich.

165.   Vegan Pepper Jack Roasted Pepper Panini

Servings: 1
Cooking Time: 4 Minutes
Ingredients:
- 2 slices bread (sourdough used)
- 2 tsp. vegan buttery spread
- 5 thin slices of tomato
- 1/4 cup (handful) of fresh basil leaves
- 1/4 - 1/3 cup vegan pepper jack cheese shreds such as Daiya
- 2-3 thin slices roasted red or yellow pepper
- 1/2 cup baby spinach
- pinches of black pepper jacklespoon Harissa

Directions:
1. Spread what's going to be the outside of each piece of bread with the vegan buttery spread. Spread the Harissas on what's going to be the inside of each piece of bread.
2. Place the tomatoes on one of the pieces of bread, then the spinach, then the basil, then the peppers, and top with the vegan cheese. Place the other piece of bread on top with the Harissa touching the cheese.
3. Cook the Panini on medium heat for 2 to 4 minutes, flipping halfway through. The bread should be brown, and the cheese should be melted.

166.   Pesto Beef And Mozzarella Panini

Servings: 4
Cooking Time: 5 Minutes
Ingredients:
- 8 slices Italian bread, 1/2 inch thick
- 2 tablespoons butter or margarine, softened
- 1/2 cup basil pesto
- 1/2 lb. thinly sliced cooked deli roast beef
- 4 slices (1 oz. each) mozzarella cheese
- Marinara sauce, warmed, if desired

Directions:
1. Spread the pesto on one side of each piece of bread. Spread the butter on the other side.
2. Split the roast beef between four pieces of bread with the pesto side up and then top with the mozzarella. Place the other piece of bread on the mozzarella with the butter side up.
3. Cook the Panini on medium heat for 5 minutes, flipping halfway through. The bread should be brown, and the cheese should be melted

167.   Veggie And Pork Mayo Sandwich

Servings: 1
Cooking Time: 3 1/2 Minutes
Ingredients:
- 1 smaller Hamburger Bun
- 1 tbsp shredded Carrots
- 1 tbsp shredded Cabbage
- 1 tbsp chopped Onion
- 1 tsp Pickle Relish
- 1 tbsp Mayonnaise
- 2 ounces chopped cooked Pork
- Salt and Pepper, to taste

Directions:
1. Grease the Hamilton Beach Breakfast Sandwich Maker with cooking spray and preheat it.
2. Cut the hamburger bun in half and brush the mayonnaise over the insides of the bun.
3. Place one of the halves inside the bottom ring, with the cut-side up.
4. Top with the pork and veggies.
5. Season with salt and pepper, and top with the pickle relish.
6. Lower the top ring and add the second half of the bun with the cut-side down.
7. Close the unit and cook for 3 ½ minutes.
8. Rotate the handle clockwise to open.
9. Transfer to a plate and enjoy!

Nutrition Info: Calories 395 Total Fats 25g Carbs 28g Protein 20g Fiber 1.5g

168.   Pepperoni Pizza Omelet

Servings: 1
Cooking Time: 4 Minutes
Ingredients:
- 2 Eggs
- 1 ounce Pepperoni, sliced
- 2 tsp Tomato Puree
- 1 ounces shredded Cheese
- Salt and Pepper, to taste

Directions:
1. Preheat and grease the sandwich maker.
2. Whisk the eggs in a bowl and season with some salt and pepper.
3. Stir in the tomato puree.
4. When the green light appears, pour half of the eggs to the bottom ring of the unit.
5. Top with the cheese and pepperoni.
6. Lower the cooking plate and the top ring, and pour the remaining eggs into the cooking plate.
7. Close and cook for 4 minutes.
8. Rotate the plate clockwise and transfer to a plate.
9. Serve and enjoy!

Nutrition Info: Calories 392 Total Fats 30g Carbs 3.2g Protein 25.6g Fiber 0.6g

169.   Portabella Havarti Melt

Servings: 1
Cooking Time: 4 Minutes
Ingredients:
- 2 slices crusty white bread
- 2 tsp. mayonnaise
- 1 tsp. Dijon mustard
- 1 portabella mushroom cap
- Spinach leaves
- 1 slice dill havarti cheese
- 1 egg

Directions:
1.   Spread mayonnaise and Dijon mustard on both slices of bread. Place one slice, mayo side up into the bottom ring of breakfast sandwich maker. Place portabella mushroom, spinach leaves and havarti cheese on top.
2.   Lower the cooking plate and top ring; crack an egg into the egg plate and pierce to break the yolk. Top with other slice of bread.
3.   Close the cover and cook for 4 to 5 minutes or until egg is cooked through. Gently slide the egg plate out and remove sandwich with a rubber spatula.

170.   Bolognese Cup

Servings: 1
Cooking Time: 3 ½ Minutes
Ingredients:
- 1 Flour Tortilla
- 2 ounces ground Beef, cooked
- 1 tsp chopped Onion
- 1 tbsp Marinara Sauce
- 1 ounce shredded Mozzarella Cheese

Directions:
1. Preheat the sandwich maker and grease it with some cooking spray.
2. Add the tortilla inside, tucking it in, until it looks like a cup.
3. Add the beef, onion, and marinara sauce inside. Stir a bit to combine.
4. Top with the shredded mozzarella cheese.
5. Close the sandwich maker and cook for 3 ½ minutes.
6. Open the lid and transfer to a plate.
7. Serve and enjoy!

Nutrition Info: Calories 375 Total Fats 24g Carbs 20g Protein 19g Fiber 1.4g

171.   Prosciutto And Pesto Panini

Servings: 4
Cooking Time: 8 Minutes
Ingredients:
- One 10-ounce loaf Ciabatta, halved horizontally and soft interior removed
- 1/3 cup Pesto
- Extra-virgin olive oil
- 1/3 pound Prosciutto de Parma, thinly sliced
- Tapenade (optional)
- 1/4 pound Fontina cheese, thinly sliced
- 1/2 cup baby arugula or basil, optional
- Coarse salt and fresh ground pepper

Directions:
1. Spread pesto on one of the interior sides and olive oil on the other.
2. Put in a layer of prosciutto, then arugula or basil, then cheese. Top it off with a light drizzle of olive oil and a sprinkle of salt and pepper. Top with the other piece of bread.
3. Brush the inside each piece of bread with the dressing. Then top the bottom pieces of bread with cheese. Add the mortadella, salami, tomatoes and pepperoncini's
4. Cook the Panini on medium-high heat for 8 minutes, flipping halfway through. The bread should be brown, and the cheese should be melted.

172.   Margherita Flatbread Mini

Servings: 1
Cooking Time: 5 Minutes
Ingredients:
- 1 round flatbread
- 1 teaspoon olive oil
- 1 clove garlic, minced
- 1 slice mozzarella cheese
- 2 thin slices ripe tomato
- 1 thin slice red onion
- 4 fresh basil leaves
- Pinch dried oregano
- 1 large egg, beaten
- 2 teaspoons grated parmesan cheese

Directions:
1. Preheat the breakfast sandwich maker.
2. Place the flatbread inside the bottom tray of the sandwich maker.
3. Brush the flatbread with the olive oil and sprinkle with garlic.
4. Add the tomatoes, red onion and basil leaves then sprinkle with dried oregano.
5. Top the vegetables with the mozzarella cheese.
6. Slide the egg tray into place and pour the beaten egg into it.
7. Close the sandwich maker and cook for 4 to 5 minutes until the egg is cooked through.
8. Carefully rotate the egg tray out of the sandwich maker then open the sandwich maker.
9. Sprinkle the sandwich with parmesan cheese then enjoy.

173.   Olive And Cheese Snack

Servings: 1
Cooking Time: 3 Minutes
Ingredients:
- 1 Bread Slice
- 1 ounce Shredded Cheese
- 1 Basil Leaf, chopped
- 2 Kalamata Olives, diced

Directions:
1. Grease the unit and preheat it until the green light appears.
2. Cut the bread slice so that it can fit inside the unit, and place it on top of the bottom ring.
3. Top with the olives, basil, and cheese.
4. Close the lid and cook for 3 minutes.
5. Rotate clockwise and open carefully.
6. Transfer with a non-metal spatula and enjoy!

Nutrition Info: Calories 205 Total Fats 12.7g Carbs 15g Protein 10g Fiber 2.1g

174.   Italian Egg Whites On Ciabatta

Servings: 1
Cooking Time: 5 Minutes
Ingredients:
- 1 ciabatta sandwich roll, sliced
- 1 teaspoon unsalted butter
- 1 slice mozzarella cheese
- 2 large egg whites
- 1 tablespoon skim milk
- 1 clove garlic, minced
- 1 teaspoon chopped chives
- 1/8 teaspoon dried Italian seasoning

Directions:
1. Preheat the breakfast sandwich maker.
2. Place half of ciabatta roll, cut-side up, inside the bottom tray of the sandwich maker.
3. Spread the butter on the ciabatta roll. Top with the slice of mozzarella cheese.
4. Whisk together the egg whites, milk, garlic, chives and Italian seasoning.
5. Slide the egg tray into place and pour the egg mixture into it.
6. Top the egg with the other half of the ciabatta roll.
7. Close the sandwich maker and cook for 4 to 5 minutes until the egg is cooked through.
8. Carefully rotate the egg tray out of the sandwich maker then open the sandwich maker and enjoy your sandwich.

175.   Turkey Bacon And Cranberry Biscuit

Servings: 1
Cooking Time: 4 Minutes
Ingredients:
- 1 store bought or homemade biscuit, sliced in half
- 1 Tbsp. canned cranberry sauce
- 2 slices turkey bacon
- 1 slice Swiss cheese
- 1 egg

Directions:
1. Spread cranberry sauce on both biscuit halves. Place one half into the bottom ring of breakfast sandwich maker, cranberry side up. Place turkey bacon and Swiss cheese on top.
2. Lower the cooking plate and top ring; crack an egg into the egg plate and pierce to break the yolk. Top with other biscuit half.
3. Close the cover and cook for 4 to 5 minutes or until egg is cooked through. Gently slide the egg plate out and remove sandwich with a rubber spatula.

176.   Sausage Omelet With Paprika And Cheese

Servings: 1
Cooking Time: 4 Minutes
Ingredients:
- 1 ounce cooked breakfast Sausage, chopped
- 2 Eggs
- 1 ounce shredded Cheese
- ¼ tsp Smoked Paprika
- 1 tsp chopped Onion
- Salt and Pepper, to taste

Directions:
1. Preheat the sandwich maker and grease it with cooking spray.
2. Whisk the eggs in a bowl and add the onion to them. Season with paprika, salt and pepper.
3. Pour half of the egg mixture to the bottom ring.
4. Top with the cheese and sausage.
5. Lower the top ring and the cooking plate.
6. Pour the remaining eggs into the cooking plate.
7. Close the unit and cook for about 4 minutes.
8. Rotate the plate clockwise and carefully open. Transfer the omelet to a plate.
9. Serve as desired and enjoy!

Nutrition Info: Calories 371 Total Fats 28.5g Carbs 2g Protein 25.5g Fiber 0.1g

177.   Beef, Waffle, And Egg Sandwich

Servings: 1
Cooking Time: 4 Minutes
Ingredients:
- 1 frozen Beef Pattie
- 2 4-inch Waffles
- 1 Egg, whisked
- ¼ tsp Garlic Powder
- Salt and Pepper, to taste
- 1 slice Cheddar Cheese

Directions:
1. Preheat the unit until the green light appears. Grease with cooking spray.
2. Add one waffle to the bottom ring.
3. Add the beef pattie on top and top with the cheddar.
4. Lower the cooking plate and add the egg to it. Season with salt, pepper, and garlic powder.
5. Close the unit and cook for 4 minutes, not less.
6. Rotate the handles clockwise, lift to open, and carefully transfer to a plate.
7. Serve and enjoy!

Nutrition Info: Calories 562 Total Fats 38g Carbs 28g Protein 38g Fiber 3g

178.   The Ham & Cheese

Servings: 1
Cooking Time: 4 Minutes
Ingredients:
- 1 English muffin, split
- Grainy mustard
- 1 slice honey spiral ham
- 1 slice cheddar cheese
- 1 egg
- Red Hot sauce

Directions:
1.   Spread some grainy mustard on both halves of English muffin. Place one half, mustard side up into the bottom ring of breakfast sandwich maker. Place ham and cheddar cheese on top.
2.   Lower the cooking plate and top ring; crack an egg into the egg plate and pierce to break the yolk. Sprinkle a few drops of Red Hot sauce on the egg and top with other muffin half.
3.   Close the cover and cook for 4 to 5 minutes or until egg is cooked through. Gently slide the egg plate out and remove sandwich with a rubber spatula.

179.   Spicy Pork And Pimento Sandwich

Servings: 1
Cooking Time: 4 Minutes
Ingredients:
- 3 ounces cooked ground Pork
- 1 ounce shredded Pimento Cheese
- 1 tbsp chopped Red Onion
- 1 smaller Hamburger Bun
- 1 ½ tsp Tomato Puree
- ½ tsp Chili Powder

Directions:
1.   Preheat the sandwich maker and grease it with some cooking spray.
2.   Cut the bun in half.
3.   When the green light appears, add half of the bun to the bottom ring.
4.   Place the pork, red onion, and cheese on top.
5.   Sprinkle the chili powder over.
6.   Lower the top ring and cooking plate.
7.   Top the sandwich with the second half with the cut-side down.
8.   Close and cook for 4 minutes.
9.   Slide out clockwise, lift it open, and transfer to a plate with a spatula that's not metal.
10.   Serve and enjoy!
Nutrition Info: Calories 532 Total Fats 28.5g Carbs 34.4g Protein 33g Fiber 1.2g

180.   Bacon Date Sandwich

Servings: 1
Cooking Time: 5minutes
Ingredients:
- 1 French Roll, split in half
- 1 tsp. Olive oil
- 2 oz. Goat cheese, soft
- 3 dates, chopped
- 4 Slices of crisp Bacon

Directions:
1. Brush the bread on the inside with olive oil.
2. On one-half place the cheese, dates, and bacon. Cover with the second half.
3. Press on the sandwich maker for 5 minutes.
4. Serve and enjoy!

181.   Pear & Greens Sandwich

Servings: 1
Cooking Time: 5 Minutes
Ingredients:
- 1 biscuit, split
- 1 Tbsp. ricotta cheese
- Pear slices
- Piece of butter lettuce
- 1 Tbsp. finely chopped walnuts

Directions:
1. Spread ricotta cheese on both biscuit halves. Place one half into the bottom ring of breakfast sandwich maker, cheese side up. Place pear slices, butter lettuce and walnuts on top.
2. Lower the cooking plate and top ring; top with other biscuit half. Close the cover and cook for 3 to 4 minutes or until sandwich is warm. Remove with a rubber spatula and enjoy!

182.   Lox And Capers Breakfast Bagel

Servings: 1
Cooking Time: 5 Minutes
Ingredients:
- 1 multigrain bagel, split
- 1 Tbsp. cream cheese
- 2 – 3 oz. lox (smoked salmon)
- Cucumber slices
- Red onion slices
- 1 ½ tsp. capers
- 1 egg

Directions:
1. Spread cream cheese on both bagel halves. Place one half into the bottom ring of breakfast sandwich maker, cream cheese side up. Place smoked salmon, cucumber slices, red onion slices and capers on top.
2. Lower the cooking plate and top ring; crack an egg into the egg plate and pierce to break the yolk. Top with other bagel half.
3. Close the cover and cook for 4 to 5 minutes or until egg is cooked. Gently slide the egg plate out. Remove sandwich with a rubber spatula and enjoy!

183.   Pepper Jack Sausage Sandwich

Servings: 1
Cooking Time: 5 Minutes
Ingredients:
- 1 buttermilk biscuit, sliced in half
- 1 tsp. horseradish sauce
- 1 pork sausage patty, cooked
- 1 slice Pepper Jack cheese
- 1 large egg, beaten

Directions:
1. Spread the horseradish sauce on the bottom half of the biscuit.
2. Preheat the breakfast sandwich maker.
3. Place the bottom half of the biscuit, cut-side up, inside the bottom tray of the sandwich maker.
4. Top the biscuit with the sausage patty and Pepper Jack cheese.
5. Slide the egg tray into place and pour the beaten egg into it.
6. Place the second half of the biscuit on top of the egg.
7. Close the sandwich maker and cook for 4 to 5 minutes until the egg is cooked through.
8. Carefully rotate the egg tray out of the sandwich maker then open the sandwich maker to enjoy your sandwich.

184.   Rotisserie Chicken Pressed Sandwich

Servings: 2
Cooking Time: 10minutes
Ingredients:
- 3 tbsp. Mayo
- 4 ½ tsp. Parmesan, grated
- 1 tsp. of Lemon juice
- ½ tsp. Pesto
- ¼ tsp. Lemon zest
- Black pepper
- 4 slices of bread, sourdough
- ¼ lb. rotisserie chicken, sliced
- 4 bacon slices, cooked fully
- 2 slices of smoked mozzarella cheese
- 4 Tomato slices
- 2 slices of red onion, separate them into rings
- 4 Tomato slices
- 2 tbsp. melted butter

Directions:
1. In a bowl, combine the mayo, Parmesan, lemon juice, pesto and lemon zest, and black pepper.
2. Spread ½ of the mixture on 2 slices of bread and layer them with tomato, onion, mozzarella cheese, bacon, and chicken.
3. Spread the remaining mayo mix over the other slices and place on top. Brush the bread with butter.
4. Cook on a sandwich maker for 4 minutes.
5. Serve and enjoy!

185.   The Ultimate Thanksgiving Reuben Panini

Servings: 4
Cooking Time: 7 Minutes
Ingredients:
- 1/3 cup mayonnaise
- 2 tablespoons cranberry sauce (I used whole berry)
- 2 teaspoons freshly grated horseradish
- 1 teaspoon Worcestershire sauce
- Kosher salt and black pepper, to taste
- 2 cups shredded green cabbage or packaged Cole slaw
- 8 slices rye bread
- 8 slices Swiss cheese
- 3/4 lb. carved turkey, thinly sliced
- 2 tablespoons melted butter

Directions:
1.   Mix together the first 4Ingredients:using a whisk. Salt and pepper to taste. Combine the mixture with the cabbage until well coated.
2.   Put a layer of cheese, then turkey, a layer of the slaw, a another layer of turkey, and another layer of cheese on a piece of bread. Top with another piece of bread. Spread the butter on the top and bottom of the sandwich
3.   Cook the sandwiches for 7 minutes on medium high heat, and make sure to flip halfway through. The bread should be toasted, and the cheese should be melted.

186.   Veggie & Cheese Melt

Servings: 1
Cooking Time: 5 Minutes
Ingredients:
- 2 slices sour dough bread
- 1 tomato slice
- 1 Tbsp. finely chopped spinach
- 1 Tbsp. finely diced precooked asparagus
- A few fresh onion rings
- 1 slice white cheddar cheese
- 1 egg
- Sea salt and pepper

Directions:
1.   Place one slice of sour dough bread into the bottom ring of breakfast sandwich maker. Place tomato, spinach, asparagus, onion and white cheddar cheese on top.
2.   Lower the cooking plate and top ring; crack an egg into the egg plate and pierce to break the yolk. Season with sea salt and pepper. Top with other slice of bread.
3.   Close the cover and cook for 4 to 5 minutes or until egg is cooked and cheese is melted. Carefully remove sandwich with a rubber spatula.

187.   Pressed Turkey Sandwich

Servings: 1
Cooking Time: 10minutes
Ingredients:
- 2 slices of bread, whole grain
- 2 tsp. Mustard
- 1/8 tsp. Rosemary, dried or fresh ¼ tsp.
- 1 grated Minutesi Cheese Round
- 2 oz. Turkey breast, smoked
- 4-5 slices of ripe pear
- Baby Spinach, a handful

Directions:
1. Preheat the Panini press.
2. Mix the mustard with the rosemary.
3. Spread the mustard on the bread slices and top one slice with turkey, ½ cheese, spinach and add the remaining cheese.
4. Put the second bread slice on top and grill on the Panini press until the cheese melts and the bread becomes golden.
5. Let it rest for 1 minutes and then serve.

188.   The Ultimate 4-minute Cheeseburger

Servings: 1
Cooking Time: 4 Minutes
Ingredients:
- 1 frozen Beef Patty
- 1 small Hamburger Bun
- 1 slice American Cheese
- 1 ounce cooked and crumbled Bacon
- 1 tsp Pickle Relish
- 2 Tomato Slices
- 1 tsp Dijon Mustard

Directions:
1. Preheat the sandwich maker and grease it with some cooking spray.
2. Cut the bun in half and place one on top of the bottom ring.
3. Add the patty on top and brush with the mustard.
4. Top with bacon, pickle relish, and tomato slices.
5. Place the cheese on top.
6. Lower the top ring and add the second bun half.
7. Close the unit and cook for 4 minutes.
8. Open carefully and transfer to a plate.
9. Serve and enjoy!

Nutrition Info: Calories 480 Total Fats 31g Carbs 24g Protein 28g Fiber 2g

189.   Cinnamon Apple Biscuit

Servings: 1
Cooking Time: 4 Minutes
Ingredients:
- 2 tbsp grated Apple
- ¼ tsp Cinnamon
- ½ Biscuit
- ½ tsp Sugar

Directions:
1. Preheat the sandwich maker and grease the insides with cooking spray.
2. Add the biscuit with the cut-side up, to the bottom ring of the unit.
3. Top with the grated apple and sprinkle the sugar and cinnamon over.
4. Close the unit and cook for 3 minutes.
5. Open carefully and transfer to a plate.
6. Serve and enjoy!

Nutrition Info: Calories 55 Total Fats 0.6g Carbs 12.2g Protein 1g Fiber 1.2g

190.   Taleggio And Salami Panini With Spicy Fennel Honey

Servings: 6
Cooking Time: 10 Minutes
Ingredients:
- 1/3 cup honey
- 1 tablespoon fennel seeds
- 2 teaspoons chili flakes
- 1/2 loaf focaccia, cut into 4-inch squares
- 1 pound Taleggio, rind washed, room temperature, thinly sliced
- 12 slices fennel salami, thinly sliced

Directions:
1. Put the chili, fennel, and honey in a small saucepan and heat on medium heat. Allow the mixture to cook for 3 to 5 minutes.
2. Cut the focaccia in half horizontally. Layer the cheese on one piece of bread and layer the salami on top. Top the salami with a nice drizzle of the honey. Put the other piece of bread on top.
3. Brush the inside each piece of bread with the dressing. Then top the bottom pieces of bread with cheese. Add the mortadella, salami, tomatoes and pepperoncini's
4. Cook the Panini on medium-high heat for 10 minutes, flipping halfway through. The bread should be brown, and the cheese should be melted.
5. Top with more honey and serve warm.

191.   Cheddar-apple Smoked Bacon Sandwich

Servings: 1
Cooking Time: 4 Minutes
Ingredients:
- 1 English muffin, split
- 1 tsp. grainy mustard
- 2 slices smoked bacon
- 3 thin apple slices
- 1 slice cheddar cheese
- 1 egg

Directions:
1.   Spread the mustard on one half of the English muffin. Place muffin, mustard side up, into the bottom ring of breakfast sandwich maker. Place smoked bacon, apple slices and cheddar cheese on top.
2.   Lower the cooking plate and top ring; crack an egg into the egg plate and pierce to break the yolk; top with other English muffin half.
3.   Close the cover and cook for 4 to 5 minutes or until egg is cooked through. Gently slide the egg plate out and remove sandwich with a rubber spatula.

192.   Goat Cheese Pesto And Egg English Muffin Panini

Servings: 4
Cooking Time: 5 Minutes
Ingredients:
- 4 egg
- 4 English muffins, split and lightly toasted
- 4 tablespoons prepared pesto
- 4 oz. Humboldt Fog goat cheese or Bucheron de chevre, sliced into 4 rounds
- 4 large tomato slices
- 8 leaves radicchio
- Olive oil
- 4 teaspoon butter

Directions:
1.   Use a whisk to beat the eggs with a pinch of salt and pepper. Place the butter in a skillet and melt it on medium heat. Use a spoon to stir the eggs and push them across the pan. Cook until the eggs set, about 1 to 2 minutes.
2.   Spread the pesto on the inside of part of the English muffins, then layer the eggs on the inside of the lower piece of the English muffin, then the cheese, then the radicchio, then the tomatoes, and top with the other half of the English muffin. Brush the top and bottom of the sandwiches with olive oil.
3.   Cook the Panini on medium heat for 4 to 5 minutes, flipping halfway through. The English muffin should be toasted, and the cheese should be melted.

193.   Lamb Panini With Thyme And Roasted Garlic Mayonnaise

Servings: 4
Cooking Time: 55 Minutes
Ingredients:
- 12 thin slices boneless, roasted leg of lamb
- 2 heads garlic
- 1/2 cup mayonnaise
- 2 tablespoons lemon juice
- 1 tablespoon fresh thyme leaves
- Salt and freshly ground black pepper
- 4 paper-thin slices sweet onion
- Fresh spinach leaves
- 1 large tomato, thinly sliced
- 4 soft sandwich rolls
- Olive oil

Directions:
1.   Preheat your oven to 375F.
2.   Use a knife to cut off the heard of the garlic cloves. Cut about ¼ inch from the top. The idea is to expose the inside of every garlic clove, and then drizzle with the oil. Bake for 45 to 50 minutes. The garlic should be sweet and soft. Allow the garlic to cool until you can handle it. Then separate the cloves from the bulb. Mash the cloves in a bowl.
3.   Mix the lemon juice, mayonnaise, and thyme with the mashed garlic until well combined. Allow it to rest for 15 minutes.
4.   Cut the sandwich rolls in half and spread the garlic mixture on the inside part of both halves of the rolls. Brush the other side of the bread with olive oil. Put a layer of onions on the bottom half of the roll, then tomatoes, spinach, and then lamb, and top with the other half of the roll.
5.   Cook the sandwiches for 5 minutes on medium heat, and make sure to flip halfway through. The bread should be nicely toasted.

194.   Feta Lamb And Babba Ghanoush Panini

Servings: 4
Cooking Time: 6 Minutes
Ingredients:
- 1 cup canned grilled eggplant pulp
- 1 small clove garlic, coarsely chopped
- 1 tablespoon tahini (sesame paste)
- 1/2 medium lemon
- Salt
- Freshly ground black pepper
- 2 to 3 sprigs flat-leaf parsley, chopped
- 8 to 12 ounces roasted leg of lamb
- 4 oval pita breads or flatbreads, cut in half horizontally
- 1 to 2 tablespoons olive oil
- 3/4 cup crumbled feta cheese

Directions:
1.   Place the eggplant, garlic, 1 teaspoon lemon juice, and tahini in a food processor. Pulse the mixture until it becomes smooth, and then salt and pepper to taste.
2.   Slice the lamb into bite sized piece. If you use pita bread use a brush to lightly coat both sides with olive oil. If you're using flatbread just coat one side.
3.   Spread the babba ghanoush spread on one side of the bread. If you're using flatbread make sure it's not the side with olive oil. Put the lamb on top of the babba ghanoush, then top with the feta, and finally sprinkle with the parsley. Top with another piece of pita or flatbread. Make sure the oil side is up if you're using flatbread
4.   Cook the sandwiches for 4 to 6 minutes on medium heat, and make sure to flip halfway through.

195.   Chili Sandwich

Servings: 1
Cooking Time: 3 – 3 ½ Inutes
Ingredients:
- 2 ounces cooked ground Beef
- 1 English Muffin
- ¼ tsp Chili Powder
- 1 tbsp chopped Tomatoes
- 2 tsp Beans

Directions:
1. Grease your Hamilton Beach Breakfast Sandwich Maker and preheat it.
2. Cut the muffin in half.
3. When the green light appears, add one muffin half with the cut-side down, to the bottom ring.
4. In a small bowl, combine the tomatoes, beans, chili powder, and beef.
5. Top the muffin half with the beef mixture.
6. Lower the top ring and add the second muffin half.
7. Close the lid and cook for 3 to 3 ½ minutes.
8. Open carefully and transfer to a plate.
9. Serve and enjoy!

Nutrition Info: Calories 320 Total Fats 16g Carbs 28g Protein 15g Fiber 3g

196.   Beans & Veggies Sandwich

Servings: 1
Cooking Time: 8 Minutes
Ingredients:
- 2 slices multigrain bread
- 2 Tbsp. canned black beans
- 2 tsp. diced green onion
- 2 tsp. shredded carrot
- 2 tsp. shredded radish
- 1 slice Pepper Jack cheese
- 1 egg
- Sea salt and pepper

Directions:
1. Spread black beans on both slices of bread. Place one slice, beans side up, into the bottom ring of sandwich maker. Sprinkle green onion, carrot and radish on top. Top with Pepper Jack cheese.
2. Lower the cooking plate and top ring; crack an egg into the egg plate and pierce to break the yolk. Season with sea salt and pepper. Top with other slice of bread.
3. Close the cover and cook for 4 to 5 minutes or until egg is cooked through. Gently slide the egg plate out and remove sandwich with a rubber spatula.

197.   Bacon & Green Chili Croissant

Servings: 1
Cooking Time: 5 Minutes
Ingredients:
- 1 medium croissant, sliced in half
- 2 tsp. mayonnaise
- 2 slices bacon
- 1 slice fresh tomato
- 1 – 2 tsp. canned diced green chilis
- 1 slice Swiss cheese
- Dash of chili powder
- 1 egg

Directions:
1.   Spread mayonnaise on both halves of croissant. Place one half in the bottom of your breakfast sandwich maker, mayo side up. Place bacon, tomato, green chili and Swiss cheese on top. Sprinkle with a dash of chili powder.
2.   Lower cooking plate and top ring. Crack an egg into the egg plate, piercing the yolk to break it. Top with other croissant half and cook for 4 – 5 minutes, or until egg is cooked through.
3.   Gently slide the egg plate out and carefully remove sandwich with a rubber spatula.

198.   Rich Flavored Sandwich

Servings: 2
Cooking Time: 5minutes
Ingredients:
- 4 slices of bread, rustic Country
- 2 tsp. Mustard
- 3 oz. (6 slices) brie
- 8 oz. Cooked ham, sliced (8 slices)
- Black pepper
- 2 tbsp. Marmalade
- 2 tbsp. Olive Oil
- ½ cup of arugula

Directions:
1.   Spread 1 tsp. Mustard on each bread slice.
2.   Layer brie and ham and season with black pepper.
3.   Spread 1 tsp. on the remaining bread slices and top the sandwich.
4.   Brush the sites with oil and place the sandwiches on the Panini grill. Cook on high until golden brown.
5.   Finish with arugula on top and serve.

199.   Fish Finger Sandwich

Servings: 1
Cooking Time: 4 Minutes
Ingredients:
- 2 Fish Fingers, cooked and chopped
- 1 small Hamburger Bun
- 1 tbsp Cream Cheese
- 1 ounce Cheddar Cheese
- 1 tbsp chopped Red Onion

Directions:
1. Preheat the sandwich maker and grease it with some cooking spray.
2. Cut the bun in half and brush it with the cream cheese.
3. Place one half on top of the the bottom ring, with the cream cheese side up.
4. Add the fish finger pieces on top, sprinkle with the red onion and top with the cheddar.
5. Lower the cooking plate and top ring and add the second half of the bun, with the cream cheese down.
6. Close the unit and cook for about 4 minutes.
7. Open carefully and transfer to a plate.
8. Serve and enjoy!

Nutrition Info: Calories 350 Total Fats 20g Carbs 26g Protein 22g Fiber 4g

200.   Spicy Horseradish Beef And Cheese Panini

Servings: 4
Cooking Time: 6 Minutes
Ingredients:
- 1/3 cup mayonnaise
- 1/4 cup crumbled blue cheese
- 2 teaspoons prepared horseradish
- 1/8 teaspoon pepper
- 1 large sweet onion, thinly sliced
- 1 tablespoon olive oil
- 8 slices white bread
- 8 slices provolone cheese
- 8 slices deli roast beef
- 2 tablespoons butter, softened
- 12 small jalapeno slices

Directions:
1. Combine the mayonnaise, blue cheese, horseradish and pepper in a bowl.
2. Sauté the onions in a skillet on medium heat until they become tender.
3. Spread the bleu cheese mixture on a single side of each piece of bread.
4. Place a layer of cheese, then jalapenos, beef, onions and then a second layer of cheese on half the pieces of bread. Place the other slices of bread on top
5. Butter the top and bottom of the sandwich and cook the Panini on medium heat for 6 minutes, flipping halfway through. The bread should be brown, and the cheese should be melted.

CPSIA information can be obtained
at www.ICGtesting.com
Printed in the USA
LVHW052234110721
692435LV00003B/26